PSYCHIATRIC
PROBLEMS

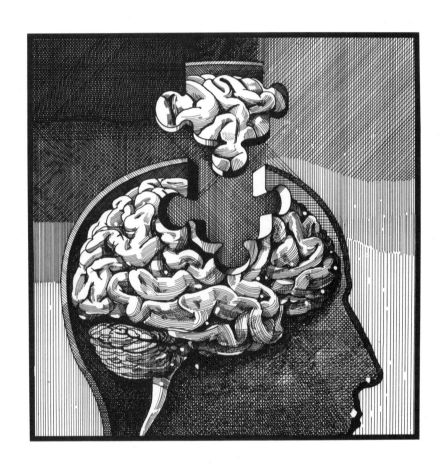

NurseReview ™

Springhouse Corporation Book Division

Chairman, Executive Board
Daniel L. Cheney

Chairman, Administrative Board
Eugene W. Jackson

President
Warren R. Erhardt

Vice-President and Director
William L. Gibson

Vice-President, Production and Purchasing
Bacil Guiley

Executive Director, Editorial
Stanley E. Loeb

Executive Director, Creative Services
Jean Robinson

Staff for this section

Editorial Director
Matthew Cahill

Clinical Director
Barbara McVan, RN

Art Director
John Hubbard

Book Editor
Michael Shaw

Editors
Catherine E. Harold, Peter Johnson, Roberta Kangilaski, Kevin Law, Edith McMahon, Pat Shapiro, Marylou Webster

Clinical Editor
Joan Mason, RN, EdM

Drug Information Manager
George J. Blake, MS, RPh

Designer
Georg W. Purvis III

Illustrators
Julia DeVito-Kruk, Robert Jackson, Robert Neumann

Production Coordination
Aline Miller (manager), Susan Hopkins Rodzewich

Editorial Services Manager
David Prout

Copy Editor
Keith de Pinho

Art Production Manager
Robert Perry

Artists
Julie Barlow, Wilbur D. Davidson

Director, Typography/Editorial CPU Services
David C. Kosten

Assistant Manager, Typography/Editorial CPU Services
Diane Paluba

Typographers
Joyce Rossi Biletz, Brenda Mayer, Robin Rantz, Brent Rinedoller, Valerie Rosenberger

Manufacturing Manager
Deborah C. Meiris

Assistant Production Manager
T.A. Landis

Production Assistant
Jennifer A. Suter

Editorial Assistants
Maree DeRosa, Beverly Lane

Clinical Consultants for this section

Brian Doyle, M.D.
Clinical Professor of Psychiatry and Family and Community Medicine Georgetown Medical School Washington, D.C.

Anna P. Moore, RN, BSN, MS
Assistant Professor and Coordinator of Psychiatric Mental Health Nursing Southside Regional Medical Center School of Nursing Petersburg, Va.

NRT12-010789

Library of Congress Cataloging-in-Publication Data

Psychiatric problems.

(NurseReview)
Includes bibliographies and index.
1. Psychiatric nursing—Handbooks, manuals, etc.
I. Springhouse Corporation. II. Series [DNLM: 1. Mental Disorders—nursing WY 160 P9736]
RC440.P774   1989   610.73'68
89-4144
ISBN 0-87434-219-8 (SC)

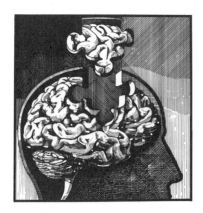

Contents

Assessment

Dysfunctional Disorders

Affective Illness

Patterns of Distorted Thinking

Destructive Coping Patterns

Cognitive Impairment

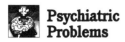

Introduction

Providing care for psychiatric patients requires that you develop a practical, orderly method for dealing with a group of disorders as diverse and complex as humanity itself. Your responsibilities include not only planning, implementing, and evaluating care but also establishing a meaningful therapeutic relationship with the patient. But because psychiatric problems are often intractable, you'll need to develop a keen awareness of your own attitudes and feelings to prevent frustration from hobbling your efforts. And you'll need to understand recent developments in neurobiology that have revolutionized treatment.

Psychiatric Problems prepares you for this challenge. Written by recognized experts, it serves as an up-to-date clinical reference that reviews assessment techniques, interventions, and nursing care measures for anxiety disorders, mood disorders, schizophrenia, delusional disorders, personality disorders, and organic mental disorders.

Throughout the book you'll find information presented according to the nursing process, outlining your role every step of the way. Sample nursing care plans help you put nursing diagnoses into action by outlining patient goals, detailing nursing interventions, and specifying outcome criteria.

The first chapter describes techniques for assessing the emotionally distressed patient. You'll find guidelines for conducting the patient interview and mental status examination. These guidelines are supplemented with advice on how to listen objectively and respond sensitively to patients, and on how to observe behavior changes that may reveal mental health problems. The chapter also provides information on diagnostic studies commonly used to evaluate psychiatric patients.

The next section begins an in-depth discussion of anxiety, a condition that rarely warrants hospitalization yet constitutes a component of almost every psychiatric disorder. After a general discussion of anxiety, you'll review specific assessment techniques and interventions for diagnosed anxiety disorders, such as phobias, panic disorder, and post-traumatic stress disorder. Included at the end of this chapter is a summary of how anxiety may affect the medical-surgical patient.

The following chapter discusses anxiety-related disorders, including dissociative, somatoform, and factitious disorders. Affected patients suffer from anxiety so overwhelming that it produces physical symptoms. Because these disorders frequently mimic organic ones, the chapter provides a careful review of assessment techniques. This review proves especially helpful because many patients derive psychological benefits from their symptoms, complicating the challenge of providing effective care.

The next chapter, on depression and bipolar disorders, is geared toward helping you increase the effectiveness of your personal interactions with the patient. You'll learn to help patients overcome loneliness, guilt, low self-esteem, and other problems. In addition, current drug therapies for mood disorders are conveniently sum-

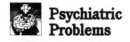
Introduction

marized in chart form. Because severe depression can lead to a suicide attempt, the chapter also discusses your role in assessing suicide potential and preventing a suspected suicide.

Next, you'll prepare for encountering the patient whose perception of reality has become grossly distorted. The chapter on schizophrenia discusses the shattering effects of this disorder and how you can help the patient achieve a more meaningful existence. You'll find up-to-date information on both neuroleptic drug therapy and psychosocial interventions. The chapter on delusional disorders will help you provide care for the patient who clings to a belief that's false but not altogether implausible.

Substance abuse, the topic of the next chapter, focuses on alcohol, opiate, and cocaine addiction. The chapter covers the range of interventions available to help these challenging patients, always emphasizing the need to deliver nursing care in a manner that doesn't communicate moral reproach. The chapter also addresses eating disorders. Like the drug-dependent patient, the patient with an eating disorder turns to an external substance—food—to solve problems; however, assessment and intervention require a vastly different approach.

The following chapter covers antisocial and borderline personality disorders. Because these patients frequently provoke strong emotional reactions, the text includes guidelines for getting in touch with your own feelings, an important part of maintaining quality care.

The final chapter discusses organic mental disorders, focusing on Alzheimer's disease and other dementias. Because many elderly persons develop dementia, the chapter outlines your role in counseling family members who witness mental deterioration in a loved one.

Concluding with references and an index, **Psychiatric Problems** promises to be an important and practical addition to your nursing library. Like all the other volumes in the NurseReview series, it provides a professional boost in today's challenging health care environment.

Assessment Techniques and Diagnostic Tests

Judith M. Saunders, an Assistant Research Scientist at the City of Hope National Medical Center in Duarté, California, co-authored this chapter. She earned her BS from the University of Cincinnati Christ Hospital School of Nursing, and her doctorate in nursing science from the University of California, San Francisco.

Co-author **Sharon M. Valente** is an Adjunct Assistant Professor of Nursing at the University of Southern California and Clinical Specialist in Mental Health in private practice. She earned her BSN at Mount St. Mary's College, Los Angeles, and is a doctoral candidate at the University of Southern California.

Psychiatric assessment refers to the scientific process of identifying a patient's psychosocial problems, strengths, and concerns. Besides serving as the basis for treating psychiatric patients, psychiatric assessment has broad nursing applications. Recognizing psychosocial problems and how they affect health is important in any clinical setting. In a medical-surgical ward, for example, you may encounter patients who experience depression, have thought disorders, or attempt suicide.

In this chapter, you'll find detailed guidelines for two major assessment techniques: the patient interview and the mental status examination. You'll also find information on observing patient behavior, assessing suicidal patients, conducting physical examinations of psychiatric patients, and diagnostic testing.

Psychiatric interview

A systematic psychiatric interview helps you acquire broad information about the patient. It includes:
- a description of the patient's behavioral disturbances
- a thorough emotional and social history
- tests of mental status.

Using this information, you'll be able to:
- assess the patient's psychological functioning
- understand coping methods and their effect on psychosocial growth
- build a therapeutic alliance that encourages the patient to talk openly
- develop a plan of care.

The success of the patient interview hinges on your ability to listen objectively and to respond with empathy. Keep in mind the following guidelines when interviewing psychiatric patients:
- Have clearly set goals in mind. Remember the assessment interview is not a random discussion. Your purpose may be to obtain information from a patient, screen for abnormalities, or to investigate further an identified psychiatric condition, such as depression, suspiciousness, or suicidal thoughts.
- Don't let personal values obstruct your professional judgment. For example, when assessing appearance, judge attire on its appropriateness and cleanliness, not on whether it suits your taste.
- Pay attention to unspoken signals. Throughout the interview, listen carefully for signs of anxiety or distress. What topics does the patient pass over vaguely? You may find important clues in the patient's method of self-expression and in the subjects he avoids.
- Take into account a patient's cultural beliefs and values. A person who blames bad luck on a power called "juju" would be considered delusional in the United States. Neighbors in Nigeria, however, would consider this quite normal. When dealing with patients from an unfamiliar culture, consult with an outside resource before making any conclusions about their psychological state.
- Don't make assumptions about how past events affected the patient emotionally. Try to discover what each event means to the patient. Don't assume, for example, that the death of a loved one provoked a mood of sadness in a patient. A death by itself doesn't

Continued on page 4

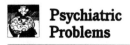

Assessment Techniques and Diagnostic Tests

Psychiatric interview—*continued*

cause sadness, guilt, or anger. What matters is how the patient perceives the loss.

• Monitor your own reactions. The psychiatric patient may provoke an emotional response strong enough to interfere with your professional judgment. A depressed patient may make you depressed and a hostile patient may provoke your anger. You may develop anxiety after an interview with an anxious patient. You may feel angry or perplexed upon encountering someone with a thought disorder. A violent, psychotic patient who has lost touch with reality may easily induce fear.

You may find yourself identifying with a patient. Perhaps the patient has similar interests or past experiences or is close to your age. Such feelings pose a real threat to establishing a therapeutic relationship; they may disrupt your objectivity or cause you to avoid or reject the patient. Consult with a psychiatric liaison nurse, doctor, or psychiatric clinical specialist if you recognize within yourself strong prejudices toward the patient. (For further information on the role of the liaison nurse, see Chapter 2.) Develop self-awareness as a tool to monitor patients and to further your own professional growth.

For further information, see *Guidelines for an effective interview.*

Interview steps

Create a supportive atmosphere. The patient must feel comfortable enough to discuss his problems. You will encounter patients who are angry and argumentative. Other patients will be too withdrawn even to say why they seek help. You will have to deal with diverse cultural norms. Some patients may come from cultural backgrounds that frown upon discussing intimate details with a stranger, even a nurse. Adolescents may refuse to discuss sexual activity in front of their parents. Listen carefully to the patient and respond with sensitivity.

Reassure the patient you respect the need for privacy. Ask privately who should be present at the interview and how the patient wishes to be addressed.

Find out the patient's purpose. Ask what the patient expects to accomplish through treatment. A person with low self-esteem may seek a better self-image. A schizophrenic may want to be rid of hallucinations. Some patients may not understand the purpose of the interview and subsequent therapy. Help such patients identify the benefits of dealing with problems openly.

Chief complaint. Ask why the patient sought treatment. Include in your assessment a statement of the chief complaint in the patient's own words. (See *Assessing the patient's chief complaint.*)

Some patients don't have a chief complaint, whereas others insist nothing's wrong. Patients enmeshed in a medical problem often fail to recognize their own depression or anxiety. Carefully observe such patients for signs of disturbed mental health.

When possible, fully discuss the patient's complaint. Ask when symptoms began, their severity and persistence, and whether they

---

Begin the interview with a broad, empathetic statement.

❝ You look distressed; tell me what's bothering you today. ❞

Explore normal behaviors before discussing abnormal ones.

❝ What do you think has enabled you to cope with the pressures of your job? ❞

Phrase inquiries sensitively to lessen the patient's anxiety.

❝ Things were going well at home and then you became depressed. Tell me about that. ❞

Ask the patient to clarify vague statements.

❝ Explain to me what you mean when you say 'they're all after me.' ❞

Help the patient who rambles to focus on his most pressing problem.

❝ You've talked about several problems. Which one bothers you most? ❞

Interrupt nonstop talkers as tactfully as possible.

❝ Thanks for your comments. Now let's move on. ❞

Express empathy toward tearful, silent, or confused patients who have trouble describing their problem.

❝ I realize it's difficult for you to talk about this. ❞

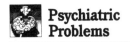
Assessment Techniques and Diagnostic Tests

Assessing the patient's chief complaint

To assess the chief complaint, ask the patient:
- What problem brought you here today?
- How long has this problem been bothering you?
- Have you or a family member had this problem before?
- When did you last feel well?

You can also assess the patient's chief complaint by interviewing family members or close friends. They may confirm behaviors that the patient may deny or clarify the complaints of confused or forgetful patients. Friends may report behavioral changes in a chemically dependent patient. Proceed with questions like these:
- When did the patient's problem begin? What led up to it?
- Has the patient been crying, become hyperactive or withdrawn, experienced changes in his sleep patterns, or exhibited any other behavior changes? When did this behavior start? How often does it occur? Does it interfere with the patient's functioning?
- What are the patient's strengths and resources?

Assessing psychological illness

To assess psychological illness and its influencing factors, ask these questions:
- What was happening in your life when symptoms first appeared?
- Who was living with you?
- Have recent events influenced the course of your illness? Has it been affected by family members?
- Do family or friends report that you behave strangely?
- What have you done to alleviate your symptoms?
- Do any activities, such as exercise, taking medication, talking, or sleeping, make the problem better? Do any activities make it worse?
- Has this problem appeared before? How was it treated?
- What else do you want to tell me?

occurred abruptly or insidiously. If discussing a recurrent problem, ask the patient what prompted seeking help at this time. To better understand the context of the illness, consider asking the questions included in *Assessing psychological illness.*

Take a psychosocial history. A psychosocial history looks at the patient's mental and social status and function. You will want to discuss the patient's beliefs, relationships, life-style, coping skills, diet, sleeping patterns, and use of alcohol, drugs, or tobacco. (See *Taking a drug history,* page 6.)

Discuss social functioning. Have the patient describe school, work, religious practices, community life, hobbies, and sexual activity.

Discuss life changes. Explore how the patient coped with such changes as a recent marriage, divorce, illness, job loss, or death of a loved one. How did the patient feel when these changes occurred?

Take a psychiatric history. Discuss past psychological disorders, such as episodes of delusions, violence, or attempted suicide. Ask if the patient has ever undergone psychiatric treatment. How did treatment help? Even though the patient may be reluctant to respond, such questions may elicit early warnings of depression, dementia, suicide risk, psychosis, or adverse medication effects.

Discuss family history. Questions about family customs, child-rearing practices, and emotional support received during childhood may reveal important insights about the environmental influences on the patient's development.

How does the patient react while disclosing family history? For example, when a patient tells you about his parents' divorce, can you detect feelings of jealousy, hostility, or unresolved grief?

Ask about the emotional health of relatives. Is there a family history of substance abuse, alcoholism, suicide, psychiatric hospitalization, child abuse, or violence? Ask about physical disorders as well. A family history of diabetes mellitus or thyroid disorders, for instance, can point to the need to investigate whether the patient's problem has an organic basis.

If the patient can't provide answers to important questions or appears unreliable, ask for permission to interview family or friends.

Discuss personal history. After clarifying the patient's chief complaint, begin a more in-depth discussion of the development of the patient's personality. Look for indications of stumbling blocks along the maturation process. (See *Major issues in development,* page 6.)

Assess the patient's ego functioning. How does the patient cope with stress? Is the patient able to control impulses and demonstrate good judgment? How strong is his sense of identity?

Don't neglect to observe areas of strength. Look for indications of the patient's adaptability, talents, accomplishments, and ability to find emotional support.

For a summary of the interview process, see *Sullivan's interview stages,* page 7.

Continued on page 8

Assessment Techniques and Diagnostic Tests

Taking a drug history

Prescription, over-the-counter, and recreational drugs may cause psychiatric symptoms, interfere with laboratory tests, reduce the effect of anesthesia, and interact with newly prescribed medications. Patients, however, may hesitate to discuss recreational drug use. Explain why you need this information and question patients directly:
- Have you ever taken nerve medications?
- What other drugs have you taken in the past?
- What medications do you take now?
- How long have you taken each one?
- How many pills a day do you take?
- Have you ever taken medications prescribed to other family members?
- If you take psychiatric or nerve medications, do you follow any special instructions regarding diet, fluids, or alcohol?
- Do you undergo lab tests regularly to monitor medication levels?
- Do drugs you take help you? What symptoms do they relieve?
- Have you noticed any adverse effects after taking drugs?
- Have you ever had tremors?
- What do you do when you forget to take your medication?
- Do you ever adjust the frequency or amount of medication you take without consulting a doctor or nurse?
- What over-the-counter or home remedies have you used?
- Have you ever used illicit drugs, such as cocaine, marijuana, or PCP? When was the last time you used them?
- Has your drug use increased during the past year?
- Have you experienced any behavior changes, such as nervousness?
- Have you ever been treated for substance abuse or addiction?
- Have you ever overdosed? If so, did you wish to harm yourself?

Major issues in development

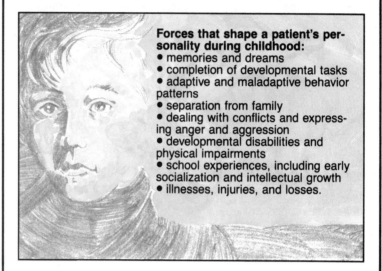

Forces that shape a patient's personality during childhood:
- memories and dreams
- completion of developmental tasks
- adaptive and maladaptive behavior patterns
- separation from family
- dealing with conflicts and expressing anger and aggression
- developmental disabilities and physical impairments
- school experiences, including early socialization and intellectual growth
- illnesses, injuries, and losses.

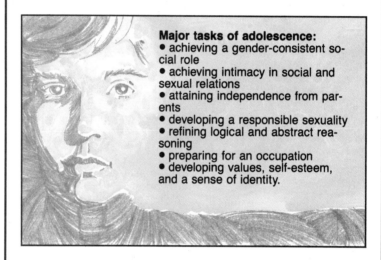

Major tasks of adolescence:
- achieving a gender-consistent social role
- achieving intimacy in social and sexual relations
- attaining independence from parents
- developing a responsible sexuality
- refining logical and abstract reasoning
- preparing for an occupation
- developing values, self-esteem, and a sense of identity.

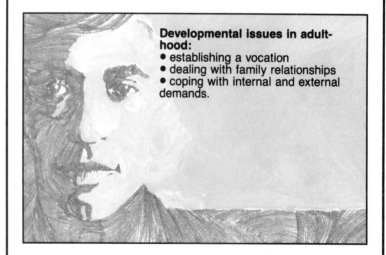

Developmental issues in adulthood:
- establishing a vocation
- dealing with family relationships
- coping with internal and external demands.

Assessment Techniques and Diagnostic Tests

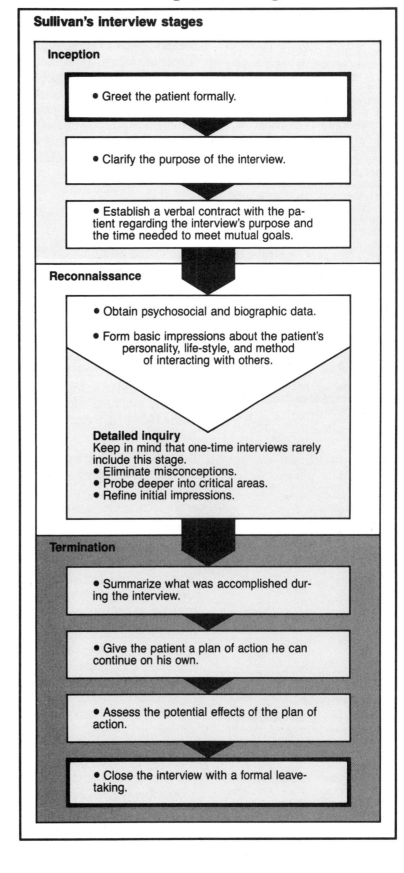

Sullivan's interview stages

Inception

- Greet the patient formally.

- Clarify the purpose of the interview.

- Establish a verbal contract with the patient regarding the interview's purpose and the time needed to meet mutual goals.

Reconnaissance

- Obtain psychosocial and biographic data.

- Form basic impressions about the patient's personality, life-style, and method of interacting with others.

Detailed inquiry
Keep in mind that one-time interviews rarely include this stage.
- Eliminate misconceptions.
- Probe deeper into critical areas.
- Refine initial impressions.

Termination

- Summarize what was accomplished during the interview.

- Give the patient a plan of action he can continue on his own.

- Assess the potential effects of the plan of action.

- Close the interview with a formal leave-taking.

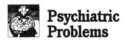 **Psychiatric Problems**

Assessment Techniques and Diagnostic Tests

Exploring risk factors

Before conducting the mental status examination (MSE), note whether the patient has a history of any psychiatric risk factors. Use the MSE to evaluate for symptoms related to these risk factors. For example, if the patient has a history of depression, examine affect, mood, and concentration during the MSE. Look for:
• past psychiatric disorders, chemical dependencies, loss of personal status, death of a loved one, psychological trauma (such as rape or incest), or physical trauma (such as a concussion or frontal lobe injury)
• family history of psychiatric disorders, such as bipolar depression or schizophrenia
• presence of an organic disorder with a psychiatric component, such as cancer (depression or anxiety), AIDS (dementia or depression), or tertiary syphilis (psychosis)
• use of drugs with psychological adverse effects, such as tranquilizers, sedatives, antidepressants, diuretics, cardiac glycosides, or antihypertensives.

Defining level of consciousness

When describing the psychiatric patient's level of consciousness, use the terms *alert, lethargic, stuporous,* or *comatose* as defined below:
• *alert*—awake, responsive, oriented to person, place, and time
• *lethargic*—diminished wakefulness; periods of excitability and irritability may alternate with periods of drowsiness
• *stuporous*—responsive only after repeated exposure to strong stimuli
• *comatose*—completely unresponsive to stimuli.

Psychiatric interview—*continued*

Mental status examination

Often included as part of the psychiatric interview, the mental status examination (MSE) is a tool for assessing psychological dysfunction and for identifying the causes of psychopathology. Understanding the components of this examination will enable you to interpret better the psychiatrist's findings as well as plan appropriate nursing interventions. Your nursing responsibilities may include conducting all or a portion of the MSE. (See *Exploring risk factors.*) The MSE examines the patient's:
• level of consciousness
• general appearance
• behavior
• speech
• mood and affect
• intellectual performance
• judgment
• insight
• perception
• thought content.

Level of consciousness. Begin by assessing the patient's level of consciousness, a basic brain function. Identify the intensity of stimulation needed to arouse the patient. Does the patient respond when called in a normal conversational tone or in a loud voice? Does it take a light touch, vigorous shaking, or painful stimulation to rouse the patient?

Describe the patient's response to stimulation, including the degree and quality of movement, content and coherence of speech, and level of eye opening and eye contact. Finally, describe the patient's actions once the stimulus is removed. (See *Defining level of consciousness.*)

An impaired level of consciousness may indicate the presence of tumor, abscess, hematoma, hydrocephalus, an electrolyte or acid-base imbalance in fluids, or toxicity from liver or kidney failure, alcohol, or drugs. If you discover an alteration in consciousness, refer the patient for a more complete medical examination.

General appearance. Appearance helps indicate the patient's overall mental status. Describe the patient's weight, coloring, skin condition, odor, body build, and obvious physical impairments. Note discrepancies between the patient's feelings about his health and your observations. Answer the following questions:
• Is the patient's appearance appropriate to his age, sex, and situation?
• Are skin, hair, nails, and teeth generally clean?
• Is his manner of dress appropriate?
• If the patient wears cosmetics, are they appropriately applied?
• Does the patient maintain direct eye contact?

A disheveled appearance may indicate self-neglect or a preoccupation with other activities. A pale, emaciated, sad appearance may indicate depression. Posture and gait may also reveal physical and emotional disorders—a slumped posture may indicate depression, fatigue, or suspiciousness, whereas an uneven or unsteady gait suggests physical abnormalities or the influence of drugs or alcohol.

Assessment Techniques and Diagnostic Tests

Assessing mood changes

Use the following guidelines when assessing a patient's mood changes:
• What are the major features of the patient's mood?
• How does this mood differ from the feelings the patient usually experiences?
• Was the onset abrupt or gradual?
• What precipitated the mood change? Look for several contributing factors.
• How intense is the mood? Is the intensity intermittent or constant?
• Has the patient experienced this mood with such intensity before? If so, what helped?
• Are the patient's mood and expression in agreement?
• How does this mood affect the patient and close friends or family members?
• As needed, assess any risks associated with a mood change. For example, assess suicide risk in patients who become depressed.

Behavior. Describe the patient's demeanor and way of relating to others. When entering the room, does the patient:
• appear sad, joyful, or expressionless?
• use appropriate gestures?
• acknowledge your initial greeting and introduction?
• keep an appropriate distance between himself and others?
• have distinctive mannerisms, such as tics or tremors?
• direct his gaze at you, at the floor, or around the room?

When responding to your questions, is the patient cooperative, mistrustful, embarrassed, hostile, or overly revealing? Describe the patient's level of activity. Is the patient tense, rigid, restless, or calm? An inability to sit still may indicate anxiety.

Note any extraordinary behavior. Disconnected gestures may indicate that the patient is hallucinating. A patient who hears voices may speak to a person who is not there and tilt his head to listen. Pressured, rapid speech and a heightened level of activity may indicate the manic phase of a bipolar disorder.

Speech. Observe the content and quality of speech, taking notice of:
• incoherency in the patient's choice of topics
• irrelevant or illogical replies
• any speech defects, such as stuttering
• excessively fast or slow speech
• sudden interruptions
• excessive volume
• barely audible speech
• altered voice tone and modulation
• slurred speech
• an excessive number of words (overproductive speech)
• minimal, monosyllabic responses (underproductive speech).

Notice how much time lapses before the patient reacts to your questions. If the patient communicates only with gestures, determine whether this is an isolated event or part of a pattern of diminished responsiveness. (For more information, see *Abnormal speech characteristics*, page 10.)

Mood and affect. Mood refers to an individual's pervading feeling tone. Usually, the patient will project a prevailing mood, though this mood may change in the course of a day. For example, depressed patients may smile occasionally but will revert to their prevailing mood of sadness. *Affect* refers to an individual's expression of his mood. Variations in affect are referred to as *range of emotion.*

To assess mood and affect, begin by asking the patient what he is feeling. Also look for indications of mood in facial expression and posture. (See *Assessing mood changes.*)

Does the patient seem able to keep mood changes under control? Mood swings may indicate a physiologic disorder. Medications, recreational drug or alcohol use, stress, dehydration, electrolyte imbalance, or disease may all induce mood changes. After childbirth and during menopause, women frequently undergo profound depression.

Continued on page 10

Assessment Techniques and Diagnostic Tests

Abnormal speech characteristics

Patients with psychiatric problems can display any number of abnormal characteristics in their speech.

Blocking

The patient loses his train of thought and stops speaking because of an unconscious block. For example, the patient may say "Well, then my mother. . . what was it I was going to say?"

Echolalia

The patient repeats the last word he hears. For example, if you say "My name is Susan," the patient responds, "Susan."

Perseveration

The patient repeats the answer to a previous question when answering a new question, despite efforts to form a new response. Perseveration also describes endless repetition of a single activity or an inability to shift from one task to another. This response usually indicates brain damage but may also signal schizophrenia.

Verbigeration

The patient repeats words, sentences, or phrases several times. This response may indicate schizophrenia. For example, a patient repeats "Now is the time. Now is the time. . . ."

Pressured speech

The patient suddenly increases the quantity of speech and becomes loud, rushed, and emphatic. This may indicate manic-depressive illness.

Neologism

The patient coins new words and endows them with a special meaning. For example, an elderly schizophrenic refers to any love object as "prattle-pie." She calls other patients as well as the pillow that she carries "prattlepie."

Flight of ideas

The patient abruptly shifts between topics that have no connection. For example, "My cat's name is Cleo. They shot the President."

Looseness of association

The patient speaks continuously and rapidly, jumping between loosely related topics. For example, "I can follow a recipe. Hindus don't eat cows. The supermarket closes at 10."

Circumstantiality

The patient describes associated ideas with too much detail, indicating a reduction in selective suppression. For example, upon being asked how his day went, a patient begins, "First I rolled on my left side. I heard the radio go off. They played a Beatles song from 1965. I thought, I hope it doesn't rain. Then I opened my eyes and could see the sun was shining. I rolled on my back and shut my eyes again. I could hear birds singing. The radio switched songs. I rolled back on my left side. . . ."

Mutism

Although capable of speaking, the patient remains silent. Mutism may indicate catatonic schizophrenia or severe depression.

Psychiatric interview—*continued*

Other symptoms of mood disorders include:
- *lability of affect*—rapid, dramatic fluctuation in the range of emotion
- *flat affect*—unresponsive range of emotion, possibly an indication of schizophrenia or Parkinson's disease
- *inappropriate affect*—inconsistency between expression (affect) and mood (for example, a patient who smiles when discussing an anger-provoking situation).

Intellectual performance. Emotionally distressed patients may show an inability to reason abstractly, make judgments, or solve problems. To develop a picture of the patient's intellectual abilities, use the

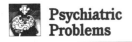 **Psychiatric Problems**

Assessment Techniques and Diagnostic Tests

Testing rote memory

The digit span
Evaluate rote memory by telling the patient a series of digits, at the rate of one digit per second, and asking him to repeat. Start by reading one to two numbers and proceed to a more difficult series of five or six numbers.

Repeat forwards:
5
3,8
4,3,1
5,7,6,3
8,3,9,2,5
3,2,9,3,5,1

Then repeat backwards:
8,5
7,2,6
4,2,3,6
7,9,2,4,5
8,7,3,6,2,1

Most adults should be able to repeat five to eight digits forward and four to six digits backward correctly. Inability to repeat five digits forward or three digits backward indicates mental impairment such as severe anxiety, dementia, or organic brain damage.

Counting and calculation
Test the patient's ability to calculate by asking him arithmetic questions appropriate to his age and education. Inability to perform simple calculations may indicate organic brain syndrome or schizophrenia.

Reading and writing
Ask the patient to read aloud from an appropriate book and to write down a piece of information, such as his address. An inability to perform these simple tasks may indicate dyslexia, dementia, or a central lesion.

following series of simple tests. Note that these tests screen for organic brain syndrome as well. If organic brain syndrome is suspected, follow up with additional physical, neurobehavioral, and psychological testing.

Orientation. Ask the patient the time, date, place, and who he is.

Immediate and delayed recall. Assess the ability of the patient to recall something that just occurred and to remember events after a reasonable amount of time.

For example, to test immediate recall, say, "I want you to remember three words: plate, glove, and bedspread. What are the three words I want you to remember?" Tell the patient to remember these words for later recall. To test delayed recall, ask the patient to repeat the same words in five or ten minutes.

Recent memory. Ask the patient about an event experienced in the past few days or hours. For example, when was he admitted to the hospital? You should know the correct response or be able to validate it with a family member. A patient may confabulate plausible answers to mask memory deficits.

Remote memory. Assess the patient's ability to remember events in the more distant past, for example, where he was born or where he attended high school. Recent memory loss with intact remote memory may indicate an organic disorder.

Rote memory. Assess the patient's ability to recall simple items without concentrated thinking. One possible test is the digit span. For further information, see *Testing rote memory.*

Attention level. You may also use the digit span to assess the ability of the patient to concentrate on a task for an appropriate length of time. Simply observe whether the patient pays attention for the length of the test. If the patient has a poor attention level, remember to provide simple, written instructions for health care.

Comprehension. Assess the ability of the patient to understand material, retain it, and repeat the content. Ask the patient to read a section of a news article and explain it.

Concept formation. To test the patient's ability to think abstractly, ask the meaning of common proverbs. Interpreting the proverb "People in glass houses shouldn't throw stones" to mean that glass is breakable shows *concrete thinking.* Interpreting the proverb as saying "Don't criticize others for what you do yourself" shows *abstract thinking.* Normally people develop abstract thinking around age 12.

Concrete answers may indicate mental retardation, severe anxiety, organic brain syndrome, or schizophrenia. Schizophrenics may also give elaborate or bizarre answers. Inability to give any answer may indicate low intellectual ability or brain damage. You may use other well-known proverbs such as "A stitch in time saves nine" or "Don't count your chickens before they hatch." Keep in mind, however, that

Continued on page 12

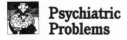

Psychiatric
Problems

Assessment Techniques and Diagnostic Tests

Psychiatric interview—*continued*

some familiar sayings may be confusing to people from foreign cultures.

Similarity tests. For another test of abstract thinking, ask the patient to describe how paired items are similar. Order pairs in increasing abstraction, for example:
• dog-horse (animals)
• mouth-nose (facial features)
• air-water (necessary for life)
• painting-poem (works of art)
• fish-tree (living objects).

An inability to recognize similarities may indicate mental retardation, schizophrenia, or dementia.

General knowledge. To determine the patient's store of common knowledge, ask questions appropriate to his age and level of learning, for example, "Who is the President?" or "Who is the Vice-President?"

Judgment. Assess the ability of the patient to evaluate choices and to draw appropriate conclusions. Ask the patient, "What would you do upon finding a stamped, addressed, sealed airmail letter lying on the sidewalk?" The answer "Track down the recipient" would indicate impaired judgment. Questions that emerge naturally during conversation (for example, "What would you do if you ran out of medication?") may also help to evaluate the patient's judgment.

Defects in judgment may also become apparent while the patient tells his history. Pay attention to how the patient handles interpersonal relationships and occupational and economic responsibilities.

Insight. Is the patient able to see himself realistically? Is he aware of his illness and its circumstances? To assess insight, ask "What do you think has caused your anxiety?" or "Have you noticed a recent change in yourself?"

Expect patients to show varying degrees of insight. For example, an alcoholic patient may admit to having a drinking problem but blame it on his work. Lack of insight may indicate a psychotic state.

Perception. Perception refers to interpretation of reality as well as use of the senses. Psychologists are placing increasing importance on perceptions in understanding psychological disorders. For example, psychoanalysts have long said that depression results from internal, unresolved conflicts that became activated after a real or perceived loss. Recently, proponents of the cognitive theory of depression have suggested that depression comes from distorted perception. Depressed patients perceive themselves as worthless, the world as barren, and the future as bleak.

Sensory perception disorders. Hallucination refers to the perception of a nonexistent external stimulus. Illusion, by contrast, refers to the misinterpretation of an external stimulus. Tactile, olfactory, and gustatory hallucinations usually indicate organic disorders.

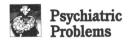
Assessment Techniques and Diagnostic Tests

Assessing hallucinating patients

To the hallucinating patient, distorted perceptions are real. A patient who hears voices will laugh at their jokes and become enraged at their insults. Because the voices are so real, you will easily be able to find out about them. Examples of questions you might ask such a patient include:
• Do you hear voices when you cannot see people?
• How many different voices speak to you?
• What do they say?
• Do you recognize the voices?
• When did you first hear voices? What else was going on in your life at that time?
• How do you respond to the voices? What gives you relief?

Not all visual and auditory hallucinations are associated with psychological disorders. For example, heat mirages, visions of a recently deceased loved one, and illusions evoked by environmental effects or experienced just before falling asleep do not indicate abnormalities. Patients may also experience mild and transitory hallucinations. Constant visual and auditory hallucinations may, however, give rise to strange or bizarre behavior. Disorders associated with hallucinations include schizophrenia and acute organic brain syndrome following withdrawal from alcohol or barbiturate addiction. (See *Assessing hallucinating patients.*)

Thought content. Assess the patient's thought patterns throughout the exam. Are the patient's thoughts well connected to reality? Are the patient's ideas clear, and do they progress in a logical sequence? Observe for indications of morbid thoughts and preoccupations or abnormal beliefs.

Delusions. Most often associated with schizophrenia, delusions are grandiose or, more commonly, persecutory false beliefs. Delusions may be obvious ("The FBI is after me"), but often their relationship with reality is ambiguous.

Obsessions. Some patients suffer intense preoccupations that interfere with daily living. Patients may constantly think about hygiene, for example. A *compulsion* is a preoccupation that is acted out, such as constantly washing one's hands. Patients often cannot control compulsive behavior without great effort.

Observe also for suicidal, self-destructive, violent, or superstitious thoughts; recurring dreams; distorted perceptions of reality; and feelings of worthlessness or persecution.

Key signs and symptoms

Besides using information from the interview and the MSE, you may assess mental health problems by observing significant changes in patient behavior. Identify departures from usual behavior patterns by comparing the results of the interview with the patient's history. Observe behavior changes that take place during the course of the assessment. When noting an important change in patient behavior, ask yourself:
• What prompted the change?
• Did the change come about slowly or abruptly?
• Is the change consistent with the patient's values, life-style, and psychological history?
• Does the change conform with societal norms?
• Does the patient show extremes in behavior or thought patterns? A change in mood may range from feeling "a little down" to feeling immobilized from depression.

Appetite. People who use food to control conflicts as well as to provide or deny themselves comfort often experience drastic changes in appetite:
• An increase in appetite may indicate anxiety.
• A decrease in appetite may warn of depression or an organic disorder such as cancer or AIDS.

Continued on page 14

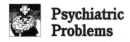

Assessment Techniques and Diagnostic Tests

Key signs and symptoms—*continued*

• Patients with *anorexia nervosa* starve themselves to remain excessively thin. To get rid of food, they may force themselves to vomit or use laxatives. Patients with *bulimia nervosa* gorge and subsequently purge themselves.

• Schizophrenic or manic patients may abruptly change their eating habits. Delusional patients may believe their food is poisoned and refuse to eat despite hunger and weight loss.

Energy levels. While energy levels normally vary, a drastic change in energy level may have its basis in an emotional disorder:

• Misdirected, extra energy may indicate anxiety.

• Excessive energy may indicate the mania of bipolar illness.

• A lack of energy, accompanied by apathy, may indicate depression. Changes in energy level may also indicate a physical disorder. Low energy levels characterize Epstein-Barr disease as well as the latter stages of chronic debilitating illness. Extra energy levels may indicate a hyperthyroid condition.

Motivation. A patient may complain about lost motivation. If such information is not forthcoming, however, inquire about interest level in his job, family, or leisure time activities. Try to determine whether the patient works toward achieving goals. Remember that goals may be very specific (getting into law school) or general (contributing to the family's well-being). Diminished motivation may indicate depression, a psychosis, or an organic disorder such as Alzheimer's disease.

Hygiene standards. A patient may become excessively concerned about cleanliness or may become very neglectful. If a patient who usually maintains personal hygiene becomes unkempt and dirty, it may signal depression, psychosis, or organic illness.

Self-image. Over time, people adapt their mental image of their appearance to accommodate the gradual changes that accompany aging. But an abrupt change in appearance, especially after an accident or colostomy, masectomy, or other surgery, may force the patient to reconcile self-image to a disturbing new reality. Some psychologists say patients with anorexia nervosa cannot reconcile their ideal with their real self-image. To assess self-image, observe how the patient responds to any abrupt body changes. Ask the patient what these changes mean, both in terms of appearance and the ability to continue activities.

Self-esteem. Does the patient place a realistic, consistent value on his own self-worth? A patient may lose self-esteem because of troubled relationships with others or a failure to live up to his own expectations. Some patients with diminished self-esteem make statements that deprecate their self-worth, minimize their abilities, and convey a lack of self-respect. Others will brag about their accomplishments, assert their own rights at other's expense, and demean others to bolster their own importance. People with low self-esteem are prone to depression and substance abuse.

Sleep. Changes in sleep habits, such as the development of insomnia or excessive sleeping, may indicate depression or anxiety. Early morning awakening and difficulty falling or staying asleep indicate depression.

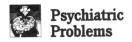
Assessment Techniques and Diagnostic Tests

Warning signs in suicidal patients

Be alert for these telltale behaviors:
- withdrawal
- social isolation
- signs of depression, which may include constipation, crying, fatigue, helplessness, hopelessness, poor concentration, reduced interest in sex and other activities, sadness, and weight loss
- long farewells to friends and family
- putting affairs in order
- giving away prized possessions
- expression of covert suicide messages and death wishes
- obvious suicide messages, such as "I'd be better off dead."

Responding to a suicide threat

If a patient shows signs of impending suicide, assess the seriousness of the intent and the immediacy of the risk. Consider a patient with a chosen method who plans to commit suicide in the next 48 to 72 hours a high risk.

Tell the patient that you're concerned. Then try to extract a promise that he will not act self-destructively until the staff has an opportunity to help him. You may specify a time for the patient to seek help.

Next, consult with the treatment team about arranging for psychiatric hospitalization or a safe equivalent, such as having someone to watch the patient at home. Initiate safety precautions before scheduling the formal psychiatric examination.

Patients may ask you to keep their suicidal thoughts confidential. Remember such requests are ambivalent; suicidal patients want to escape the pain of life, but they also want to live. A part of them wants you to tell other staff so they can be kept alive. Tell patients that you can't keep secrets that endanger their lives or conflict with their treatment. You have a duty to keep them safe and to ensure the best care.

Sexual drive. Changes in sexual drive provide valuable information in psychological assessment, but you may have to sharpen your skills in assessing sexual activity. Prepare yourself for patients who are uncomfortable discussing their sexuality. Avoid language that implies a heterosexual orientation. Introduce the subject tactfully but directly. For example, begin by saying "I'm going to ask you a few questions about your sexual activity because it's an important part of most everyone's life."

Follow-up questions might include:
- Are you currently sexually active?
- Do you usually have relations with men or women?
- Have you noticed any recent changes in your interest in sex?
- Do you have the same pleasure from sex now as before?
- Do you understand safe sex guidelines? Do you think your sexual practices are safe?

Competence. Is the patient still able to understand reality and the consequences of his actions? Does the patient understand the implications of his illness, its treatment, and the consequences of avoiding treatment? Use extreme caution when assessing changes in competence. Unless behavior strongly indicates otherwise, assume the patient is competent. Remember that legally only a judge has the power or right to declare an individual incompetent to make decisions regarding personal health and safety or financial matters.

Assessing self-destructive behavior

Healthy, adventurous people may intentionally take death-defying risks, especially during youth. The risks taken by self-destructive patients, however, are not death-defying but death-seeking.

Suicide refers to intentional, self-inflected death. Suicide may be carried out with guns, drugs, poisons, rope, automobiles, or razor blades, or by drowning, jumping, or refusing food, fluid, or medications. In a *subintentional suicide,* a person has no conscious intention of dying but nevertheless engages in self-destructive acts that could easily become fatal.

Not all self-destructive behavior is suicidal in intent. Some patients engage in self-destructive behavior because it helps them to feel alive. A patient who has lost touch with reality may cut or mutilate body parts to focus on physical pain, which may be less overwhelming than emotional distress. Such behavior may indicate a borderline personality disorder.

Assess depressed patients for suicide. (See Chapter 2.) Not all of them want to die, but a higher percentage of depressed patients commit suicide than patients with other diagnoses. Chemically dependent and schizophrenic patients also present a high suicide risk.

Suicidal schizophrenics may become agitated instead of depressed. Voices may tell them to kill themselves. Alarmingly, some schizophrenics provide only vague behavioral cues before taking their lives.

Upon perceiving signals of hopelessness, perform a direct suicide assessment. (See *Warning signs in suicidal patients.*) Protect patients from self-harm during a suicidal crisis. After treatment, patients will think more clearly and, hopefully, find reasons for living.

Continued on page 16

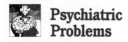
Assessment Techniques and Diagnostic Tests

Physical examination

Because psychiatric problems may stem from organic causes or medical treatment, doctors often order a physical examination for psychiatric patients. Observe for key signs and symptoms and examine the patient by using inspection, palpation, percussion, and auscultation. (For more complete information on physical examination, see the "Patient Assessment" chapters in NURSEREVIEW.)

Cranial nerves

A defect in perception may indicate a disturbance in one or more of the cranial nerves. A neurologic assessment will help to determine whether a sensory defect results from a damaged or dysfunctioning nerve or a conversion disorder. For example, a patient may complain of sudden paralysis of one hand. A neurologic assessment would indicate that the nerves are intact, thereby indicating a conversion disorder.

Cerebellar function. The cerebellum controls equilibrium and muscle function to assure smooth, steady, and coordinated movement. Cerebellar dysfunction can result from several causes, including cerebellar degeneration or tumor and Parkinson's disease.

Abnormal findings may include:
- *intention tremors*—Rhythmic, involuntary movement of voluntary muscles that increases with voluntary activity
- *cerebellar ataxia*—an unsteady gait that forces the patient to keep his legs wide apart when standing
- *cerebellar nystagmus*—abnormal rhythmic movements of the eye
- *adiadochokinesia*—an inability to perform rapid alternating movements.

An abnormality in cerebellar function may cause the patient to become dependent on other people and mechanical devices for simple tasks such as walking, bathing, or cooking. Children with cerebellar abnormalities may have few opportunities to play because of their inability to perform simple maneuvers. Patients may experience intense loneliness, sadness, or feelings of uselessness.

Sensory system

The sensory system carries impulses from the various areas of the body to the central nervous system (CNS), which registers and interprets them. Perceived sensations include simple touch, pain, temperature, stereognosis, two-point discrimination, and the extinction phenomenon.

Abnormal sensations include:
- *anesthesia*—complete loss of ability to perceive stimuli
- *hypoesthesia*—reduced sensory perception
- *hyperesthesia*—increased sensory perception
- *paresthesia*—abnormal sensation such as tingling
- *dysesthesia*—abnormal noxious or painful sensation.

If a sensation disorder occurs along the distribution pathway of a nerve, chances are it is organically based. Otherwise, suspect a somatoform disorder. In hysterical anesthesia, for example, the loss of sensation may involve only one extremity. Above a defined line, sensation is normal. With each examination, patients with somatoform disorders may complain of a different area and degree of sensation loss.

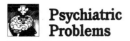
Assessment Techniques and Diagnostic Tests

Patients experiencing a sensory disturbance will likely undergo severe psychological stress, becoming at once demanding and withdrawn. Patients who experience a grief reaction may lose interest in personal grooming.

Motor system

Neurons carry impulses from the cerebrum to the skeletal muscles through the pyramidal and the extrapyramidal motor tracts. Impulses traveling along the *pyramidal tract* stimulate individual muscles; those traveling along the *extrapyramidal tract* stimulate groups of muscles. The upper motor neuron tracts extend from the cerebrum to the anterior horn motor neurons. The lower motor neuron tracts extend from the anterior horn motor neurons to the skeletal muscles.

When assessing the motor system, observe muscle tone, size, and strength. Distinguishing signs and symptoms help to identify whether an injury occurred to an upper or lower motor neuron tract.

Symptoms of an upper motor neuron tract disturbance include:
• hyperreflexia below the area of the disturbance
• pathologic reflexes
• hypertonicity of large groups of muscles
• no fasciculations
• mild muscular atrophy
• slightly decreased muscle strength.

Symptoms of lower neuron tract disturbance include:
• absence of reflexes below the area of disturbance
• absence of pathologic reflexes
• hypotonicity confined to specific muscle groups
• fasciculations
• severe muscular atrophy
• absence of muscle strength
• abnormal gait (organic disturbance).

The symptoms of motor disturbances associated with somatoform disorders include tics, tremors, and various paralyses. All such patients show disturbed motor function with no apparent physiologic change. (See *Comparing conversion reaction and organic paralysis*, page 18.)

Seizures. When dealing with psychiatric patients, distinguishing between organically based seizures and psychogenic seizures, feigned to gain attention or prescription medication, presents great difficulty. Generally, positive differentiation requires telemetry and EEG results as well as determination of prolactin levels, which rise during organically based seizures. (For further information, see *Comparing psychogenic and tonic-clonic seizures*, page 19.)

Diagnostic studies

Diagnostic studies performed on psychiatric patients include the dexamethasone suppression test, standard laboratory tests, noninvasive studies, brain imaging studies, and psychological tests.

Dexamethasone suppression test

The dexamethasone suppression test (DST), a standardized and easily performed indirect measurement of cortisol hyperactivity,

Continued on page 18

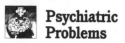 **Psychiatric Problems**

Assessment Techniques and Diagnostic Tests

Comparing conversion reaction and organic paralysis

Assessment	Conversion reaction paralysis	Organic paralysis
Muscle wasting	No appreciable muscle wasting	Appreciable muscle wasting
Muscle paralysis	Proximal muscle paralysis is greater than that of peripheral muscles	Peripheral muscle paralysis is greater than that of proximal muscles
Forearm position	Extended	Moderately flexed
Deep tendon reflexes	Present in flaccid forms	Absent in flaccid forms

Diagnostic studies—*continued*

serves as a diagnostic test for depression and a research tool in suicide studies.

In this procedure, the patient receives a 1-mg dose of corticosteroid (dexamethasone). Normally, the pituitary stops producing adrenocorticotropic hormone (ACTH), which sends a message to the adrenal glands that adequate cortisol is in the system. Cortisol levels normally stay very low for about 18 hours. Many depressed patients, however, continue to produce cortisol. The presence of normal or high blood cortisol levels provides supportive evidence for depression.

Standard laboratory tests
The purposes of running standard laboratory screening tests on psychiatric patients include:
• ruling out systemic infection; cardiovascular, endocrine, or neurologic disorders; or diseases such as syphilis and tumors.
• establishing normal kidney and liver function to assure safe absorption and excretion of psychotropic medications. If not adequately metabolized or excreted, psychotropic medications commonly cause cardiac dysrhythmias, increased blood sugar level, and toxic effects. Lithium, for example, may quickly become toxic or lethal. Tricyclic antidepressants may increase blood sugar and cause cardiac abnormalities.
• detecting signs and symptoms of disease that psychologically distressed patients may be unaware of or deny.

Urinalysis. The doctor will order a routine urinalysis to evaluate kidney function and dehydration. Before placing a patient on psychotropic drugs, kidney and liver function should be evaluated. Cautiously observe patients who take psychotropic drugs if urinalysis is abnormal. Many of these drugs are excreted in the urine; if not eliminated properly, levels will become toxic, causing tachycardia, tremors, or urinary retention.

Teach your patients how to collect a clean catch, midstream specimen. If possible, have the patient collect the first morning urine specimen. To avoid contamination, instruct a menstruating patient to insert a fresh tampon before collecting the specimen. If she doesn't

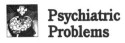
Assessment Techniques and Diagnostic Tests

Comparing psychogenic and tonic-clonic seizures

Assessment	Psychogenic seizures	Tonic-clonic seizures
Pupils	Normal	Fixed and dilated
Repirations	Possibly rapid	Temporarily interrupted, then occurring with muscle contractions. May be stertorous
Muscle contractions	Irregular	Forceful, rhythmic
Response to pain	Possible	None
Bowel and bladder function	Usually not incontinent of urine	Urinary and fecal incontinence

use tampons, consider postponing the urinalysis until after menstruation.

Send the specimen to the laboratory as soon as possible or follow proper storage protocol. Standing at room temperature causes the specimen to become alkaline, dissolves cellular elements, and increases bacterial growth.

Glucose. In addition to routine urinalysis, you may test for glucose and ketones in the urine using a reagent strip. Normally the glomeruli filter glucose out and the proximal tubules absorb it. However, psychotropic drugs may induce borderline glycosuria.

Patients with hyperglycemia develop pathologic glycosuria if blood glucose levels exceed the patient's renal threshold (generally about 170 mg/dl.) Stress, pregnancy, or consumption of high-carbohydrate foods may induce transient nonpathologic glycosuria. High urine glucose levels may also indicate diabetes mellitus, renal glycosuria, or Fanconi's syndrome.

Proteins. Because proteins are too large to pass through the glomerular capillaries, they normally don't appear in the urine. However, albuminaturia and proteinuria may occur in alcoholic patients. Transient proteinuria may follow stress, exposure to cold, or fever. Chronic proteinuria may indicate severe infection or renal disease.

Hematologic studies. A complete blood count (CBC) helps evaluate kidney function and detect diseases that may cause psychiatric symptoms, such as infection, anemia, or tumors.

Hemoglobin and hematocrit. Normal hemoglobin values range from 12 to 16 g/dl for women and from 14 to 18 g/dl for men. Normal hematocrit values range from 37% to 47% for women and 45% to 57% for men.

Elevated hemoglobin and hematocrit levels indicate dehydration. Dehydration may induce hypovolemia, aggravate dementia, or lead to delirium in elderly or debilitated patients. Decreased hemoglobin and hematocrit levels may indicate acute renal disease, cancer, or fluid overload.

Continued on page 20

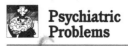
Assessment Techniques and Diagnostic Tests

Diagnostic studies—*continued*

Red blood cell (RBC) count. Normal values for RBC count differ according to age and sex. Normal values for men range from 4.5 to 6.2 million/mm³; for women, from 4.2 to 5.4 million/mm³; and for children, from 4.6 to 4.8 million/mm³. An increased RBC value may indicate dehydration or primary or secondary polycythemia. Secondary polycythemia is characteristic of chronic obstructive pulmonary disease patients and alcoholics. A decreased RBC value may signal fluid overload, recent hemorrhage, or anemia. Anemia may follow any chronic systemic disease.

White blood cell (WBC) count. Normal values for WBC count range from 4,100 to 10,900/mm³. An elevated WBC value may indicate infection associated with increased catabolism and subsequent protein breakdown. Toxic effects on the brain may lead to acute confusion.

Psychotropic drugs can cause aplastic anemia, agranulocytosis, thrombocytopenia, and leukopenia. All these conditions are serious, making early detection of hematologic changes urgent. Be alert for fever, sore throat, mouth ulcers, easy bruising, or hemorrhage. Instruct patients to report these signs immediately.

Tegretol, which raises the seizure threshold and helps in treating bipolar illness, bears a hematologic risk. As ordered, measure CBC and platelet count before the patient begins taking the drug, then monitor monthly for the next 6 months.

Electrolytes. Characteristic of alcoholics, fluid and electrolyte disturbances often disrupt mental status. Commonly measured electrolytes include:

Serum sodium. An abundant cation, sodium helps the kidneys regulate body fluid. Consequently, sodium levels are evaluated in relation to the amount of body fluid. Normal serum levels range from 135 to 156 mEq/liter. High levels may occur with dehydration, excessive salt ingestion, or excessive fluid loss. Low levels result from excessive salt loss through the kidneys or excessive water intake. Lithium use combined with a low-salt diet may also cause low sodium levels, because lithium therapy often results in polydipsia.

Serum potassium. A cation, potassium is the most abundant intracellular electrolyte. Serum levels normally range from 3.5 to 5 mEq/liter. Changes in adrenal steroid hormone secretion as well as fluctuations in pH, serum glucose, and serum sodium affect potassium levels. Expect to find low potassium levels in patients with anorexia nervosa.

Serum chloride and bicarbonate. An anion, chloride is most abundant in extracellular fluid. Normal levels range from 98 to 106 mEq/liter. Chloride levels relate inversely to bicarbonate levels. To help maintain the blood's osmotic pressure, either a chloride or a bicarbonate ion accompanies each sodium ion reabsorbed in the renal tubules. To preserve acid-base balance, when bicarbonate levels fall, the kidneys conserve chloride, thereby causing chloride levels to rise. In alcoholic patients, expect to find elevated chloride levels associated with renal disease and metabolic acidosis. Excessive

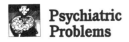
Assessment Techniques and Diagnostic Tests

vomiting and loss of hydrochloric acid leads to hypochloremic alkalosis in anorexic patients.

Serum calcium and phosphorus. Calcium levels normally range from 4.5 to 5.5 mEq/liter; phosphorus levels, from 1.8 to 2.6 mEq/liter. Calcium and phosphorus have an inverse relationship: when one rises, the other falls. To maintain balance, parathyroid hormone controls renal tubular reabsorption or excretion of phosphorus.

In hypercalcemia, the parathyroid glands increase calcitonin secretion, thereby inhibiting bone absorption and subsequent calcium release.

Blood glucose. Elevated levels may indicate diabetes mellitus or a renal disorder. Normal levels vary according to the testing method. For guidance, check your hospital's laboratory manual.

Thyroid function tests. Although most psychiatric patients have normal thyroid function, doctors routinely order thyroid studies, including triiodothyronine (T_3) and thyroxine (T_4) levels and the free thyroxine index, to rule out a thyroid disorder as a cause of mental distress. Doctors may also order thyroid studies before patients receive lithium to monitor for hypothyroidism.

Liver function tests. Serum glutamic-oxaloacetic transaminase (SGOT) and serum glutamic-pyruvic transaminase (SGPT) levels are routinely measured to determine if the liver adequately detoxifies medications. Expect to find abnormal test results in alcoholic patients. Look for symptoms of mental illness in toxic patients.

Syphilis tests. Commonly associated with psychiatric disorders, tertiary syphilis causes irreversible dementia.

Serologic tests to screen for syphilis include the Venereal Disease Research Laboratories (VDRL), rapid plasma reagin (RPR), and fluorescent treponemal antibody (FTA) tests.

Well standardized and widely used, the VDRL is a flocculation test employing nontreponemal antigen. The test becomes reactive 6 weeks after initial contact with the infecting organism, 2 to 3 weeks after a chancre appears. Positive results may be further described as weakly reactive or reactive. To monitor response to treatment, a quantitative measurement reports the last dilution for which the patient's serum is reactive.

As ordered, follow up with an RPR or FTA test if you suspect a false-positive result or have reason to question nonreactive VDRL results.

Human immunodeficiency virus (HIV) testing. Because AIDS can cause psychiatric complications, you may have to test for human immunodeficiency virus (HIV) infection. HIV-infected patients commonly suffer dementia and depression, often before revealing other significant symptoms. Dementia is one of the illnesses diagnostic of AIDS.

Psychiatric complications associated with HIV infection may result from opportunistic infections, neoplasms, or from direct action of HIV on the CNS.

Continued on page 22

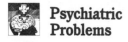
Assessment Techniques and Diagnostic Tests

Toxicology screening

The list below indicates whether toxic levels can be detected in blood, urine, or both.

Blood

alcohol (ethyl, isopropyl, and methyl)
ethchlorvynol (Placidyl)

Urine

alphaprodine (Nisentil)
chlorpromazine (Thorazine)
cocaine
desmethyldoxepin (metabolite of doxepin)
heroin (metabolized to and detected as morphine)
imipramine (Tofranil)
methadone
morphine
phencyclidine

Both

acetaminophen
amitriptyline (Elavil)
amobarbital (Amytal)
butabarbital (Butisol)
butalbital (Fiorinal)
caffeine
carisoprodal (Soma)
chlordiazepoxide (Librium)
codeine
desipramine (Pertofrane)
desmethyldiazepam (metabolite of diazepam)
diazepam (Valium)
diphenhydramine (Benadryl)
doxepin (Sinequan)
flurazepam (Dalmane)
glutethimide (Doriden)
ibuprofen (Motrin, Advil)
meperidine (Demerol)
mephobarbital (Mebaral)
meprobamate (Miltown, Equanil)
methapyrilene
methaqualone (Quaalude)
methyprylon (Noludar)
norpropoxyphene
nortriptyline (Aventyl)
oxazepam (Serax)
pentazocine (Talwin)
pentobarbital (Nembutal)
phenobarbital (Luminal)
propoxyphene (Darvon)
salicylates and their conjugates
secobarbital (Seconal)
talbutal (Lotusate)

Diagnostic studies—*continued*

Expect to use the enzyme-linked immunosorbant assay (ELISA) and the Western blot tests to detect HIV antibodies. Tests now under development may allow direct detection of the virus.

Blood will usually be drawn, though both tests will work with samples of body tissues and other fluids, such as cerebrospinal fluid (CSF). If the ELISA is positive, expect to use the more precise and expensive Western blot test to confirm results. Doctors consider positive results on the Western blot test evidence of HIV infection even in the absence of clinical symptoms.

Before testing, make sure the patient understands the test and has given informed consent to the doctor. When assisting with testing, follow the Centers for Disease Control guidelines for universal body fluids. Provide adequate support and counseling for patients who are HIV-positive and safeguard confidentiality of test results.

Toxicology screening. Screening the blood or urine may detect drugs present in concentrations greater than 5 μg/ml. With current methods, you may quantitate drugs detected in the blood only. (For further information, see *Toxicology screening*.)

When psychiatric patients receive drug therapy, expect to monitor levels to make sure the patient is not receiving a toxic dose. For example, lithium carbonate has a small therapeutic range. Absorption rates and serum levels will vary among patients. Draw blood when the concentration of serum lithium is stable, either immediately before the next dose of lithium or 8 to 12 hours after the last dose. Effective levels of lithium range from 1 to 1.5 mEq/liter. At concentrations higher than 1.5 mEq/liter, lithium becomes toxic, possibly resulting in coma or death.

Noninvasive studies

Expect the patient to receive:
- a chest X-ray and EKG to screen for heart and pulmonary abnormalities
- an EEG to screen for brain abnormalities, especially if the patient is taking psychotropic medications.

Explain each procedure to your patient beforehand.

Brain imaging studies

Computed tomography (CT) scan. A CT scan combines radiology and computer analysis of tissue density (as determined by dye absorption) to study intracranial structures. This test can help detect brain contusion or calcifications, cerebral atrophy, hydrocephalus, inflammation, and space-occupying lesions, such as tumors, hematomas, edema, and abscesses. It can also help detect vascular changes, such as arteriovenous malformations, infarctions, blood clots, and hemorrhages.

Magnetic resonance imaging (MRI). This test takes advantage of certain cell nuclei that magnetically align, and then fall out of alignment, after radio-frequency transmission. In a process called precession, the MRI scanner records signals from nuclei as they realign; it then translates the signals into detailed pictures of body

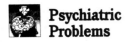
Assessment Techniques and Diagnostic Tests

structures. Compared with conventional X-rays and CT scans, MRI provides superior contrast of soft tissues, allowing sharp differences of healthy, benign, and cancerous tissue as well as clear images of blood vessels. It also allows imaging of multiple planes, including direct sagittal and coronal views, in regions where bones usually interfere.

In CNS studies, MRI can detect structural and biochemical abnormalities associated with many conditions, including transient ischemic attacks (TIAs), tumors, cerebral edema, and hydrocephalus.

Positron emission tomography (PET) scan. Unlike CT scans, which show organ structure and tissue density, PET scans provide colorimetric information about the brain's metabolic activity by detecting how quickly tissues consume radioactive isotopes. This allows direct visualization of brain functioning, including cerebral blood flow, oxygen use, and aspects of glucose metabolism.

PET scans can help detect cerebral dysfunction associated with seizures, TIAs and stroke syndromes, head trauma, and some mental illnesses. They also help evaluate the effects of neurosurgery and drug therapy and may eventually be used to confirm brain death. Currently, however, few hospitals can afford the expensive PET scanning equipment or the cyclotron that manufactures isotopes, so PET scan use is largely confined to research.

Magnetoencephalography (MEG). An experimental technique mapping the brain's electrical activity, MEG promises to improve neurologic diagnosis and treatment. MEG uses a superconducting quantum interference device to measure the brain's magnetic field. This extremely sensitive instrument takes measurements at different points on the scalp and converts the data into a color contour brain map.

Researchers have used MEG primarily to guide surgery by locating epileptic seizure foci and spread patterns. Other possible future uses include:
● identifying the origin of parkinsonian tremors
● differentiating Alzheimer's disease from other dementias
● determining brain function after a stroke or head trauma
● localizing cortical lesions responsible for vision defects
● analyzing the effects of drugs on the CNS
● investigating the mechanisms involved in memory, selective attention, and psychiatric disorders
● illuminating the brain's functional organization.

Topographic brain mapping (TBM). A new computerized technique, TBM makes EEG findings easier to interpret. To discern patterns from multiple parallel EEG tracings, the doctor must try to correlate the tracings spatially and temporally. TBM removes such obstacles by quantifying and graphically displaying EEG data. Instead of tracings, TBM displays a map on a computer-controlled video screen. By interpolating values, the computer generates contour lines with colors corresponding to each variable's intensity. Consequently, TBM allows clearer identification of certain patterns, particularly hemispheric asymmetry.

Continued on page 24

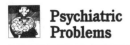

Assessment Techniques and Diagnostic Tests

The Rorschach test

The illustration depicts two of ten inkblots which patients are shown during a Rorschach test. The patient describes his impressions upon seeing each inkblot and the psychologist analyzes the content of the responses as an aid in personality evaluation.

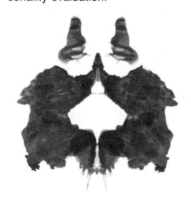

Diagnostic studies—*continued*

Doctors use TBM to:
- evaluate seizure disorders, subtle sensory deficits, psychiatric and learning disorders, and certain dementias
- diagnose regrowth of glioblastoma
- monitor brain activity in patients undergoing anesthesia or other procedures affecting brain activity
- assess the effects of drug therapy.

Psychological tests

The final component of mental health assessment, psychological tests provide information you will incorporate in your care of mentally distressed patients. To measure intelligence, psychologists administer individual, oral tests consisting of a verbal and a performance section. Such tests include Stanford-Binet test, Wechsler Adult Intelligence Scale (revised), and Wechsler Intelligence Scale for Children (revised).

Personality and projective tests elicit a patient response that provides insight into psychopathology, mood, or personality. Through the indirect approach of these tests, the patient projects his inner self. Popular personality and projective tests include the Beck Depression Inventory, the Minnesota Multiphasic Personality Inventory, the Rorschach test, the sentence completion test, the draw-a-person test, and the thematic apperception test.

Beck Depression Inventory (BDI). A self-administered, self-scored test, the BDI asks patients to rate how often they experience symptoms of depression, such as poor concentration, suicidal thoughts, guilt feelings, and crying. Questions focus on both cognitive symptoms, such as impaired decision-making, and on physical symptoms, such as loss of appetite. Elderly and physically ill patients commonly score high on questions regarding physical symptoms; their scores may stem from aging, physical illness, or depression.

The sum of 21 items gives the total, with a maximum score of 63. A score of 11 to 18 indicates mild depression. More than 18 indicates moderate depression.

You may help patients complete the BDI by reading the questions, but be careful not to influence their answers. Instruct patients to choose the answer that describes them most accurately.

If you suspect depression, a BDI score above 11 may provide objective evidence of the need for treatment. To monitor the patient's depression, repeat the BDI during the course of treatment. Consider administering a BDI to colleagues who appear depressed or burnt out and to yourself when you sense the onset of depression.

The Minnesota Multiphasic Personality Inventory (MMPI). A structured paper-and-pencil test of 566 items, the MMPI provides a practical technique for assessing personality traits and ego functioning in adolescents and adults. Most patients who read English will require little assistance in completing the test.

Psychologists translate a patient's answers into a psychological profile. Use caution in interpreting profiles. Patient answers are

Assessment Techniques and Diagnostic Tests

compared with diagnostic criteria established and standardized in the 1930s. Critics charge that the personality profile models developed in the 1930s were based on studies of small groups (30 people) and may no longer provide a valid basis for diagnosis. For example, no one has revised the outdated 1930s standards for measuring aggressive sexual impulses. Psychologists who strictly adhere to MMPI criteria would incorrectly evaluate adolescents raised under today's more permissive standards as excessively aggressive.

Test results include information on coping strategies, defenses, strengths, gender identification, and self-esteem. The psychologist compares the patient's profile with data gathered from the interview and explains the test results to the patient.

A patient's test pattern may strongly suggest a diagnostic category. If results indicate a suicide risk or high potential for committing violence, monitor the patient's behavior. If they show frequent somatic complaints indicating possible hypochondria, evaluate the patient's physical status. If complaints lack medical confirmation, help the patient explore how these symptoms may signal emotional distress.

Sentence completion test. The patient completes a series of partial sentences. A question might read, "When I get angry, I . . . ."

Draw-a-person test. The patient draws a human figure of each sex. The psychologist interprets the drawing systematically and correlates his interpretation with diagnosis. The draw-a-person test also provides an estimate of a child's developmental level.

Thematic apperception test. Upon seeing a series of pictures that depict ambiguous situations, the patient tells a story describing each picture. The psychologist evaluates these stories systematically to obtain insights into the patient's personality, particularly regarding interpersonal relationships and conflicts.

Self-test

1. To assess the patient's rote memory, ask him to name his birth place.
a. true   **b.** false

2. When interviewing a patient, observe for changes in all of the following areas except:
a. energy levels   **b.** sleep patterns   **c.** hormone levels   **d.** personal hygiene

3. Like computed tomography scans, positron emission tomography scans reveal organ structure and tissue density.
a. true   **b.** false

Answers (page number shows where answer appears in text)
1. **b** (page 11)   2. **c** (page 14)   3. **b** (page 23)

Anxiety Disorders: Generalized Anxiety, Panic, and Other Problems

Barbara Gross Braverman, a psychotherapist in private practice in Philadelphia, Pa., wrote this chapter. She earned her BSN from Temple University in Philadelphia and her MSN from Wayne State University in Detroit, Mich.

Although few patients undergo hospitalization for anxiety, a clear understanding of this common complaint will help you deal effectively with large numbers of distressed patients. That's because you'll encounter anxiety as a component of almost every psychological disorder and many organic diseases as well.

This chapter focuses on diagnosed anxiety disorders, such as phobias, panic disorder, and post-traumatic stress disorder. After reviewing anxiety's many aspects, the chapter explores anxiety in a hospital setting.

Aspects of anxiety

Closely related to fear, anxiety nevertheless constitutes a distinct emotional state. Fear, by definition, is an acute response to a clearcut external threat, whereas anxiety is a diffuse response to a vague threat. Anxiety affects all of us at some point in our lives. Generally, people experience anxiety as a feeling of worry, insecurity, apprehension, or foreboding. Such feelings may represent a short-term emotional reaction or may persist and strongly shape personality development.

Each person seeks some form of expression for anxiety, both consciously and unconsciously. (See *Understanding defense mechanisms.*) Participating in sports or maintaining a busy schedule enables many to cope. However, an overly anxious person may seek to protect his beleaguered sense of self through various maladaptive defense mechanisms, such as developing somatoform pain symptoms, withdrawing from social life, or overindulging in drugs or alcohol.

Anxiety and maladaptive coping mechanisms may damage mental well-being. When anxiety and inner conflict become overwhelming, a psychiatric disorder develops. Its nature depends on how much anxiety a person suffers.

Anxiety is difficult to pinpoint because it touches upon many different aspects of human life. One way to better understand anxiety is to consider individually its physical, emotional, intellectual, social, and spiritual aspects.

Physical aspects. Through stimulation of the autonomic neuroendocrine and cardiovascular systems, anxiety causes perspiration, palpitations, and flushed face. When the patient faces a threat, anxiety may cause blood flow to shift away from the viscera and skin and toward the heart, muscles, and brain, preparing the patient for fight or flight. Anxiety states may produce fight or flight responses, though the flight response is more commonly associated with acute fear. (See *Comparing responses to anxiety and fear,* page 28.)

In the *fight response,* induced by sympathetic stimulation, blood pressure and heart and pulse rate rise. The extremities turn cold, with tremors and shivering. Hands and feet become sweaty. Pupils dilate, increasing visual acuity. Bronchial passages enlarge, allowing greater oxygen intake to meet the increased metabolic rate. Epinephrine production also rises, causing the liver to convert glycogen to glucose for increased energy. The reaction may inhibit peristaltic action, gastric secretion, and salivation.

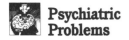 **Psychiatric Problems**

27 Dysfunctional Disorders
Anxiety Disorders

In the *flight response,* induced by parasympathetic stimulation, blood pressure and heart rate decline, and skin and visceral blood vessels dilate. Pupils narrow, and digestive processes accelerate. The changes may cause gastric distress, diarrhea, and urinary urgency. The slowed heart rate, reduced blood pressure, and decreased muscle tone may cause fainting.

Anxious patients exhibit physiologic responses in many situations, even between bouts with stress, and often take a long time to return to normal functioning. Observation of these responses will help guide your nursing diagnosis and intervention.

Emotional aspects. Anxiety is linked to various emotions, including guilt, grief, and anger. Especially significant is the connection between *guilt* and anxiety. Guilt involves a personal struggle that

Continued on page 28

Understanding defense mechanisms
Defense mechanisms help to relieve anxiety. They include conversion, denial, and many others.

Conversion
Symbolic expression of intrapsychic conflict through physical symptoms that help channel and control unbearable feelings.

Denial
Disowning intolerable thoughts, wishes, deeds, and facts to escape unpleasant realities.

Compensation
Attempting to make up for real or perceived deficiencies by concentrating on developing other abilities. Emphasizing one activity helps to relieve fear of failure In another. Overcompensation may lead to development of a one-sided personality.

Displacement
Redirecting an emotional feeling from the appropriate person or object to a less-threatening person or object. Displacement allows a safe release of feelings.

Dissociation
Separation and detachment of an idea or situation from its emotional significance. Dissociation helps an individual put aside painful feelings.

Fantasy
Consciously creating a mental image that expresses fears, wishes, and needs. Fantasy provides a symbolic means to release unacceptable thoughts and solve conflicts.

Identification
Attempting to refashion oneself in the image of an admired, idealized person. Identification preserves the ego while disguising inadequacies.

Internalization
Taking within and symbolically incorporating external wishes, values, and attitudes.

Projection
Attributing to others aspects of one's self, such as intolerable wishes, feelings, and motives, to avoid awareness of one's own undesirable impulses.

Rationalization
An attempt to make unacceptable feelings and behavior acceptable to the ego. Rationalization helps maintain self-respect and prevent guilt feelings.

Reaction formation
Assumption of attitudes and behavior that one consciously rejects. This is a protective device to avoid expressing painful or unacceptable attitudes.

Regression
Retreating to an earlier and more comfortable level of adjustment. Regression causes an individual to become more dependent and consequently less anxious.

Repression
Involuntarily submerging unbearable ideas and impulses to the unconscious realm. Repression protects the ego from guilt, shame, or lowered self-esteem.

Restitution
Attempting to assuage unconscious guilt feelings by offering others some kind of reparation.

Sublimation
Diversion of unacceptable instinctual drives into personally and socially acceptable areas to help channel forbidden impulses into constructive activities.

Substitution
Replacing an unacceptable need, attitude, or emotion with one that is more acceptable. By disguising motives, substitution helps reduce frustration.

Suppression
Intentional exclusion of forbidden ideas and anxiety-producing situations from the conscious level.

Undoing
Actually or symbolically removing a previous action or experience that has become intolerable. Undoing represents an attempt to repair feelings or actions that have created guilt or anxiety.

Anxiety Disorders

Comparing responses to anxiety and fear

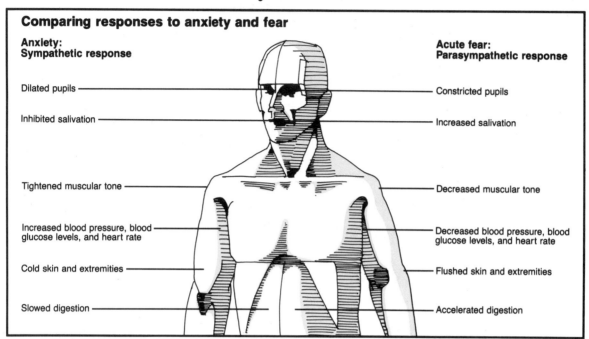

**Anxiety:
Sympathetic response**

Dilated pupils

Inhibited salivation

Tightened muscular tone

Increased blood pressure, blood glucose levels, and heart rate

Cold skin and extremities

Slowed digestion

**Acute fear:
Parasympathetic response**

Constricted pupils

Increased salivation

Decreased muscular tone

Decreased blood pressure, blood glucose levels, and heart rate

Flushed skin and extremities

Accelerated digestion

Continued

usually induces feelings of anxiety. For instance, a young child may develop guilt and anxiety when struggling to deal with hostile feelings toward his parents. An adult may experience guilt as he becomes increasingly aware of discrepancies between his actual and ideal self. Freud, recognizing this connection, identified guilt as moral anxiety.

Guilt-induced anxiety may be related to the fear of punishment. A guilt-ridden person usually fears punishment, but wants to be punished as well. Anxiety may also develop following efforts to repress guilt-provoking memories or attitudes. Interestingly, guilt may produce physiologic responses similar to anxiety, such as heavier breathing, chest heaviness, muscular laxity, slowed gait, and stooped posture.

Closely linked to guilt, *shame* refers to anxiety over being thought unworthy. Sullivan identifies shame as social anxiety. Both shame and guilt can cause a person to forsake important interpersonal support.

Grief forms another important component of anxiety. It occurs in response to the loss of a loved one or other source of emotional satisfaction. *Anger* may occur in protest to loss. A child first behaves angrily when his parents try to restrict his behavior. Venting his angry feelings helps him cope with anxiety.

Intellectual aspects. As with other emotions, a person's perceptions largely influence his anxiety level. When aroused physiologically, a person will interpret his feelings according to experience. For example, a person may interpret increased heart rate, rapid breathing, and trembling as joy or anger, depending on how he perceives precipitating events.

Anxiety Disorders

Continued on page 30

Signs of anxiety

Intellectual anxiety
- Anticipation of unpleasantness
- Blocking of words
- Difficulty concentrating
- Excessive vigilance
- Feelings of helplessness, confusion, and being restrained
- Focusing on details
- Habitual responses
- Inability to learn or reason
- Indecisiveness
- Lack of awareness of surroundings
- Loss of short-term recall
- Narrowed sensory perception
- Overreacting to stimuli
- Preoccupation with anxious feelings
- Selective inattention
- Sense of impending catastrophe
- Unrealistic thinking
- Worry over outcome of events

Social anxiety
- Apprehension when with groups of people
- Attention-seeking behavior, such as crying
- Aversion of gaze
- Blaming of others for anxiety-producing situations
- Demanding behavior
- Desire to be left alone
- Fear of losing control in social situations
- Feelings of forlornness, sadness, loneliness, shyness, or uncertainty
- Frequent touching
- Irritation or coldness with close friends and family
- Seeking to communicate with others
- Stammering or slips of speech
- Talkativeness or extreme quietness
- Withdrawal or aggression

Spiritual anxiety
- Alienation from others
- Fear of death, failure, or the future
- Feelings of hopelessness, guilt, and despair
- Inability to cope, love, or find meaning in life
- Indifference to previously important things
- Lack of belief in the future
- Lack of sense of free choice
- Rejection of long-held beliefs
- Resistance to change
- Withdrawal

An anxious person usually perceives some future unpleasantness; the dreaded event is about to happen or may happen, but it isn't happening now. However, a person experiencing anxiety after a traumatic event such as rape, combat, or a close brush with death doesn't share this future orientation. The anxiety response occurs when the person remembers the event and reexperiences it through flashbacks.

Distorted perceptions may increase anxiety. A person may work himself into a cycle—a threatening thought produces anxiety, which makes the threat seem worse and produces more anxiety. He becomes preoccupied with himself, and his self-doubt increases while self-esteem diminishes.

Anxious preoccupations interfere with rational thought, and the patient's reactions become irrelevant and self-centered. For example, an overly anxious patient may overhear you discussing preparations for a blood transfusion and immediately believe the procedure is for him, even though he is about to be discharged. An overly anxious patient will respond with apprehension to virtually any situation, and will learn complex tasks very slowly.

Social aspects. Social anxiety refers to discomfort caused by tense social situations. The socially anxious person doesn't fear personal harm or attack but becomes highly disturbed by other people's scrutiny or remarks. He has low self-esteem and fears rejection.

A socially anxious person may withdraw if others ignore him or pay too much attention. He responds shyly to remarks calling attention to aspects of his appearance. Conspicuousness, novelty, and fear of evaluation all contribute to the experience of social anxiety. He may become anxious upon overhearing private conversations or witnessing private acts, or he may fear disclosing too much personal information.

Job loss, retirement, loss of a close friend or relative, illness, new living conditions, reduced financial status, or decreased independence may induce social anxiety. Other causes include influences from highly anxious family members or friends, lack of social support, inability to meet others' expectations, and inability to have one's own emotional needs met.

Spiritual aspects. Religious faith and commitment to moral values deflect despair and provide a sense of purpose and motivation for living. The values one holds become important sources of support when confronted with illness or death. Anxiety may become severe for people undergoing intense spiritual conflicts. Such conflicts may take many forms: a loss of faith in long-cherished beliefs, a lack of personal fulfillment, guilt over a transgression of moral standards, a need for greater autonomy and self-expression, inability to receive or give love, fear of death, development of an identity crisis, or deep-rooted fear of failure.

People discard old values and adopt new ones as part of normal growth and during emotional crises. This growth process can generate anxiety. (See *Signs of anxiety.*)

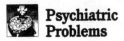
Anxiety Disorders

Continued

Classifying anxiety

Pathologic expressions of anxiety have long been defined as *neuroses.* However, definitions of neuroses, derived from loose groupings of symptoms, have led to many disagreements in diagnosis. What's more, not all doctors and psychologists agree with the theory behind the concept of neurosis.

To avoid these difficulties, the revised third edition of the American Psychiatric Association's *Diagnostic and Statistical Manual of Mental Disorders* (DSM-III-R) classifies psychiatric disorders based on observation of symptoms, using three categories: anxiety, somatoform, and dissociative disorders. (See Chapter 3 for discussion of the latter two categories.) Anxiety disorders include generalized anxiety disorder, panic disorder, phobic disorders, obsessive-compulsive disorder, and post-traumatic stress disorder.

Generalized anxiety disorder

Anxious patients don't usually present an overt psychiatric problem because they can function in most circumstances, are oriented to reality, and demonstrate no major affective disturbance. Symptoms are usually not severe enough to warrant hospitalization.

Emotional symptoms. Besides feeling upset and apprehensive, patients are often tense, irritable, and emotionally drained. They may have impaired perceptions of other people, situations, and of the meaning of events, which they interpret in ways that explain and justify their feelings. Generally, people will ignore anxious feelings so long as they don't interfere with daily activities. However, if the discomfort produced by anxiety persists or worsens, many will decide to seek help.

Depressed mood and flat affect may accompany anxiety. However, depressive symptoms are secondary complaints; the mood disturbance doesn't affect the patient's life and activities as much as the anxiety symptoms.

Physical symptoms. These may include chest pain, cold clammy hands, diarrhea, dizziness, dry mouth, dyspnea, faintness, increased pulse and blood pressure, nausea, palpitations, perspiration, and trembling. In addition, patients may describe restlessness, fatigue, muscular aches, and insomnia. In patients with generalized anxiety disorder, physical symptoms persist for at least 1 month.

Social symptoms. Anxiety adversely affects social function. As symptoms worsen, marital and family relationships undergo strain. Some patients begin to fail at work or school. Many, however, continue to fulfill their social responsibilities.

The physical symptoms of anxiety may provide the patient with acceptable reasons for altered social functioning. They allow the patient to gain added support from friends and family and to be relieved of expected activities and responsibilities. However, keep in mind that the patient doesn't have voluntary control over these symptoms.

Anxiety Disorders

Assessment

Your assessment may depend largely on the patient's own description of his feelings of uneasiness or interruptions in daily living. Ask the patient what caused him to seek treatment. Further exploration of the patient's responses will reveal more precisely the nature of his problem. Questions like "What happened that caused you to lose your job?" may encourage the patient to express himself.

Note if the patient is apprehensive about his physical symptoms. He may complain of breathing difficulty or choking, or assert that he's having a heart attack. When physical symptoms are acute, you'll need to reduce his anxiety level before attempting an interview. Reassure him that help is available. If needed, have him walk the hallway and breathe into a paper bag to combat hyperventilation and help him regain control.

Because of autonomic stimulation, physical symptoms of anxiety mimic a variety of physical illnesses, including cardiac impairment, pulmonary embolus, stroke, and hyperthyroidism. To distinguish symptoms of anxiety from those of potentially serious illness, conduct a thorough health examination.

Question the patient about alcohol and substance abuse. Patients frequently use drugs and alcohol to try to allay feelings of anxiety. Perhaps 25% of people with anxiety disorder are heavy drinkers, and 15% are alcohol-dependent. Note that early symptoms of alcohol withdrawal, including shakiness, perspiration, upset stomach, insomnia, and increased pulse rate, mimic anxiety symptoms.

Distinguishing anxiety from depression. Symptoms more indicative of depression include persistent dysphoria, psychomotor retardation, diurnal variation, early morning awakening, suicidal thoughts, and a sense of hopelessness. Patients with an anxiety disorder report autonomic hyperreactivity, perceptual distortions, derealization, and anxious impatience rather than hopelessness. Such patients may not have lost interest in their usual activities, but have lost the ability to perform them satisfactorily.

Cognitive symptoms. Expect to find only minimal cognitive impairment. The patient should be able to tell you the date, his name, and other basic personal information. However, as anxiety worsens, his perception may become distorted, and his ability to process information may become impaired. Severe anxiety, in fact, can prompt thought blocking, in which the patient can't complete a sentence or phrase. If the patient's thinking seems tangential, rambling, or circumstantial, assess for panic attacks or phobic reactions.

Thought patterns. Assess for thoughts that indicate somatic complaints, feelings of anxiety, phobic reactions, or obsessions. Although a patient may seem delusional about certain themes, particularly the meaning of somatic symptoms and phobic reactions, such beliefs aren't true delusions because the patient knows the thoughts are irrational. Less common are such symptoms as suicidal and homicidal ideation, defensive thinking patterns, hallucinations, and illusions.

Continued on page 32

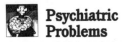
Anxiety Disorders

Generalized anxiety disorder—*continued*

Diagnostic studies. Blood studies may show increased adrenal function, elevated glucose and lactic acid levels, decreased calcium and oxygen levels, and diminished parathyroid function. Urine studies may show increased epinephrine and norepinephrine levels.

Planning

Before determining your nursing care plan, develop the nursing diagnosis by identifying the patient's actual or potential problem, then relating it to its cause. Possible nursing diagnoses for a patient with anxiety include the following:
- anxiety; related to an intangible threat or conflict
- coping, ineffective individual; related to increased feeling of conflict secondary to severe anxiety
- thought processes, altered; related to inability to make decisions secondary to anxiety
- communication, impaired (verbal); related to severe anxiety
- self-esteem, disturbance in; related to severe anxiety
- social interaction, impaired; related to lack of support network
- social isolation; related to impaired communication
- spiritual distress; related to withdrawal from usual religious practices
- comfort, altered (decreased pain perception); related to severe anxiety
- mobility, impaired physical; related to tense, rigid muscles secondary to anxiety.

The sample nursing care plan below shows expected outcomes, nursing interventions, and discharge planning for one nursing diagnosis listed. You'll want to tailor each care plan to fit your patient's needs.

Intervention

Intervention focuses on reducing anxiety and preventing it from developing into panic. To accomplish this goal, the patient may undergo behavioral therapy, psychotherapy, drug therapy, or a combination of these treatments.

Behavioral therapy. This type of therapy aims to modify the patient's behavior rather than resolve the internal conflicts and unconscious

---

Sample nursing care plan: Generalized anxiety disorder

Nursing diagnosis	Expected outcomes
Coping, ineffective individual; related to increased feelings of conflict secondary to severe anxiety	The patient will: • reduce his anxiety level. • develop healthy coping techniques.

Nursing interventions	Discharge planning
• Provide a calm, comfortable environment. • Discuss patient's behavior with him. • Encourage patient to explore the threat or conflict. • Accept patient's thoughts and feelings. • Help patient explore previously successful coping mechanisms. • Help him develop new coping skills.	• Review effective coping mechanisms with patient and family. • Consult with community psychiatric specialist to provide follow-up as necessary. • Refer patient and family to a self-help group.

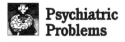
Anxiety Disorders

How desensitization works

Systematic desensitization can help overcome a patient's anxieties through gradual exposure to the phobic stimulus. Consider the patient who fears flying and seeks profesional help. His therapy might take place in these sequential "sessions":

> The patient drives to the airport, turns around, and goes home.

> Next, he takes another trip to the airport, but parks his car and sits in the visitors' lounge.

> During the following session, the patient walks to the boarding area.

> Next, he sits in the cockpit of the airplane for several minutes.

> Following this, he sits in a first-class passenger seat for a few minutes.

> During the next session, he sits in a passenger seat in the coach section for about an hour.

> Then, while sitting in the plane, the patient carries on a conversation with the flight attendant.

After several more sessions, the patient is able to take a short domestic flight.

processes causing discomfort. Common techniques include systematic desensitization and operant conditioning.

In *systematic desensitization*, the therapist teaches the patient to relax while exposing him to an anxiety-producing situation. First the patient is exposed to the mildest, least anxiety-provoking stimulus. As he progresses in therapy, he's exposed to increasingly stronger stimuli until he can tolerate the most extreme stimuli without eliciting symptoms. (See *How desensitization works.*) In *operant conditioning*, the therapist teaches the patient to correct his behavior by providing rewards for producing the appropriate response.

Relaxation exercises can be used to calm the patient before systematic desensitization. Guided imagery, accompanied by controlled breathing, helps the patient use his imagination to redirect his attention and reduce his anxiety level. These techniques may also help patients cope with stress.

Psychotherapy. Supportive psychotherapy allows the patient to express his feelings in a safe environment and encourages positive behavior. *Insight-oriented therapy* focuses on comprehending and resolving the internal conflict thought to produce the anxiety. Psychotherapy may be combined with drug therapy for more effective treatment.

Drug therapy. Such therapy may relieve the patient's anxiety symptoms and help him cope long enough to interact usefully with his therapist and others. Different drugs offer a wide range of action. The doctor may order a drug with fast onset for maximum impact, slow onset to minimize sedation, short action to allow rapid clearing, or long action to minimize rebound symptoms after treatment or between doses. When a patient begins drug therapy, warn him to avoid activities requiring alertness and neuromuscular coordination until the central nervous system (CNS) effects of the drug have been determined. (See *Selected drugs for treating anxiety*, page 34.)

Doctors frequently order *benzodiazepines* to treat generalized anxiety. Benzodiazepines reduce anxiety without the sedation caused by barbiturates and nonbarbiturate sedative-hypnotic agents. In addition, overdose and acute withdrawal less frequently result in morbidity and mortality.

Expect to administer low doses at first and titrate upwards. Dosages vary, but for most cases of generalized anxiety, they rarely exceed 30 mg of diazepam (or its equivalent) daily. Inform patients that drug therapy will be of limited duration and will diminish, but not eradicate, their symptoms. For persistent anxiety, patients may benefit most from anxiolytics during exacerbations. Other patients report sustained improvement with maintenance treatment. Monitor length of time drug is given. Long-term therapy may cause psychological and physical dependence.

Depending on the dose and treatment duration, withdrawal syndrome may follow if the drug's stopped abruptly. Usually, patients experience only mild symptoms, but some suffer severe withdrawal.

Continued on page 34

Anxiety Disorders

Selected drugs for treating anxiety

Drug and usual oral dosage	Adverse effects	Special considerations
alprazolam (Xanax) 0.25 mg to 0.5 mg t.i.d.	Anorexia, bitter taste, central nervous system (CNS) depression, coma, confusion, constipation, dry mouth, hiccups, increased appetite, somnolence	• Do not administer for depressive neuroses or psychotic reactions without anxiety.
buspirone hydrochloride (BuSpar) Initially, 5 mg t.i.d.	Diarrhea, dizziness, drowsiness, dry mouth, fatigue, headache, insomnia, nausea, nervousness	• Before initiating buspirone therapy in patients who are taking benzodiazepines, warn against stopping benzodiazepines abruptly, to avoid a withdrawal reaction.
chlordiazepoxide hydrochloride (Librium) 5 to 25 mg t.i.d or q.i.d.	Abdominal discomfort, blurred vision, constipation, decreased libido, drowsiness, fainting, hangover, hypotension (transient), lethargy, nausea, vomiting	• Use cautiously in patients with chronic pulmonary disease.
clonazepam citrate (Rivotril) 1 to 4 mg daily, given in morning and bedtime doses.	Abnormal eye movements, abnormal thirst, ataxia, behavioral disturbances, change in appetite, confusion, constipation, drowsiness, eosinophilia, gastritis, leukopenia, nausea, rash, respiratory depression, slurred speech, thrombocytopenia, tremor, urinary dysfunction	• Never withdraw drug suddenly. • Efficacy hasn't been fully evaluated. Typically used as an anticonvulsant.
clorazepate dipotassium (Tranxene) 7.5 to 60 mg daily in divided doses.	Blurred vision (occasional), confusion, constipation, depression, euphoria, singultus	• Observe patient for mood changes. • Monitor elimination.
diazepam (Valium) 2 to 10 mg b.i.d. to q.i.d.	Ataxia, drowsiness, fatigue, nightmares, sleep disturbances, weakness	• Note any changes in patient's sleep or behavior patterns. • Investigate complaints of skin, muscle, or localized pain.
hydroxyzine hydrochloride (Atarax) 25 to 100 mg every 4 to 6 hours as needed.	Bradycardia, diarrhea, dry mouth, increased gastric motility, transient drowsiness. Antiemetic reaction with increased appetite may induce weight gain.	• Observe patient's elimination patterns and weight. Start diet plan to maintain normal pattern if necessary. • Provide ice chips or mints for dry mouth. • Increases sedative effects of opiates and barbiturates.
oxazepam (Serax) 10 to 30 mg t.i.d. or q.i.d.	Abdominal discomfort, agranulocytosis, drowsiness, fainting, hangover, jaundice, lethargy, nausea, vomiting	• Use cautiously in patients with a history of convulsive disorders, drug allergies, blood dyscrasias, renal disease, or depression. • Severe withdrawal symptoms may occur.
propranolol hydrochloride (Inderal) 10 mg q.i.d.	Arthralgia, bradycardia, congestive heart failure, diarrhea, fatigue, fever, hallucinations, hypoglycemia (without tachycardia), hypotension, increased airway resistance, lethargy, nausea, peripheral vascular disease, vivid dreams, vomiting	• Always check patient's apical pulse rate before giving drug. If you detect extremes in pulse rate, hold medication and call the doctor immediately. • Efficacy has not been established. Used on an investigational basis to treat anxiety. Some doctors consider propranolol an acceptable second-line agent when benzodiazepines fail.

Generalized anxiety disorder—*continued*

Patients receiving usual doses for less than 4 months face a much lower risk of withdrawal. Expect to discontinue treatment gradually, tapering doses according to patient response.

Keep in mind that the sedative effects of benzodiazepines enhance those of other CNS depressants and that use with certain other drugs, such as cimetidine, will increase plasma levels. Also keep in mind that some patients taking higher-potency benzodiazepines may exhibit increased hostility, aggressiveness, and fits of rage.

Some doctors may order low doses of *neuroleptics* for anxiety-ridden patients who show no signs of accompanying psychosis or delirium.

Anxiety Disorders

Such drugs may have a helpful tranquilizing effect, but akathisia or other neuroleptic effects may obscure benefits. Expect to restrict use of neuroleptics to days, or weeks at most, because the availability of other effective treatments outweighs the risk of tardive dyskinesia.

Beta blockers, such as propranolol, may alleviate peripheral autonomic symptoms, such as tremors and tachycardia, but prove less effective against worry, panic attacks, or other cognitive symptoms. Patients who experience fatigue or dysphoria with propranolol may use agents that cross the blood-brain barrier less easily, such as atenolol. Effective doses vary. Expect to titrate upward from low initial doses.

Buspirone, an anxiolytic agent, calms without the sedative or additive CNS depressant effects of other drugs. Researchers have yet to determine whether buspirone works against panic attacks or severe acute anxiety, but it appears adequate for milder forms of distress. When given in doses roughly equivalent to those normally used in diazepam therapy, buspirone doesn't cause withdrawal symptoms. However, it may not benefit patients who've previously received benzodiazepines.

Researchers are testing the efficacy of *antidepressants* in generalized anxiety unassociated with panic or depression. Recent studies indicate that tricyclic antidepressants, such as imipramine, diminish persistent anxiety, though less rapidly than other common anxiolytics.

Nursing care measures. Begin by helping to identify the source and symptoms of the patient's anxiety. After identifying its source, help relieve discomfort by providing emotional support. Speak in a calm voice, using short, comprehensible sentences.

Make supportive statements that communicate kindness, warmth, and honesty. You might say, for example, "You are trying very hard, keep up the good work," or "I can see that you're improving." Touch the patient gently to reassure him, but be firm with an indecisive patient. To avoid increasing the patient's anxiety and fear, remember to control your own expression of anxiety.

The patient with acute anxiety feels too much and thinks too little. Try moving him to a calm, quiet environment to reduce stimulation. Ask questions and make observations that encourage him to use his intellect. To help him feel secure, tell him "You're safe here."

Encourage the patient to talk. Allow him to lead the discussion, but ask relevant questions. If he can express himself with clear, descriptive statements, he'll achieve a healthful release of feelings. If the patient has difficulty stating feelings, you'll need to slow down the conversation. Use facial expression to encourage the patient's involvement and indicate you are listening. Keep in mind that insensitive comments may escalate the patient's anxiety into panic.

If the patient's anxiety diminishes considerably, encourage him to recognize and deal with conflict. If his conflicts are severe, he'll

Continued on page 36

Anxiety Disorders

Helping to ease anxiety

Using simple, practical techniques, you may be able to provide immediate relief to patients suffering from anxiety.

Exercise

Encourage the patient to engage in activities such as walking, jogging, swimming, calisthenics, or yard work. Exertion uses large motor muscles, allows the patient to safely discharge excess tension and energy, and enables the patient to focus on simple, concrete tasks. Activities can be performed alone or with others.

Relaxation and meditation

Teach the patient relaxation and meditation exercises. First, ask the patient to begin by taking deep, slow, cleansing breaths. Next, have the patient tense each major muscle group for 10 seconds and then relax. Instruct him to systematically tense and relax each major group in rotation until the whole body is relaxed. Encourage the patient to do relaxation exercises on his own.

After doing the relaxation exercises, the patient is usually relaxed enough to be able to meditate. Encourage the patient to visualize something positive and soothing, such as the ocean, a sunset, a color, a wave pattern, or a loved one. Instruct the patient to concentrate on the image for 10 to 15 minutes. Meditation further releases tension and is emotionally soothing. Once the patient learns relaxation and meditation techniques, he can apply these techniques whenever anxiety and tension begin to build.

Changing the environment

Encourage the patient to rearrange his living quarters to reduce anxiety. This can be accomplished by reducing external stimuli and using soft sounds and calming colors, such as blue, green, and beige. Providing soft (but not shadowy) lighting helps to reduce visual distortion. Encourage the patient to avoid bright-colored paintings, murals, or posters. If hospitalization is needed, assign the patient to a room sheltered from the noise and bustle of the hospital unit, yet not isolated from others, if possible. The patent shouldn't have a roommate who is manic, loud, interfering, or disruptive.

Generalized anxiety disorder—*continued*

need counseling to deal with the meaning of symptoms, recurring stress, and past experiences.

Cognitive techniques. Use a problem-solving approach to uncover the patient's fears, concerns, and anxieties. An anxious patient may feel better after hearing a clear, honest statement of fact about his situation than if given a tranquilizer. He may feel relieved, for example, to know that he's experiencing stress and not the effects of a damaging illness. A hyperventilating patient may benefit from hearing his symptoms are reversible.

By watching his own interactions over time, the patient may be able to distinguish his own patterns of behavior in anxiety-producing situations. Encourage him to recognize and use this ability. Help the patient to discover gaps in his self-knowledge that may either contribute to anxiety or prevent its relief. (See *Helping to ease anxiety.*)

Evaluation

Base your evaluation on the expected outcomes listed on your nursing care plan. To determine whether your patient's improved, ask yourself these questions:
- Does the patient appear less anxious?
- Are his coping mechanisms healthy?

Your answers will help you evaluate your patient's status and the effectiveness of his care. Keep in mind that these questions stem from the sample care plan on page 32. Your questions may differ.

Other anxiety disorders

Panic disorder

Panic disorder refers to a sudden, intense feeling of apprehension, terror, and impending doom. Panic attacks represent anxiety at its most intense and leave the patient shaken, fearful, and exhausted. Most attacks last only a few minutes, although rarely they may continue for hours. Typically, patients can't tolerate panic attacks for a long time. As a result, they may seek help or develop maladaptive defensive mechanisms, such as projection.

At least four symptoms of anxiety accompany each panic attack. Episodes involving less than four symptoms are called limited symptom attacks. They sometimes progress to the full panic syndrome, but may also be disabling in their own right and lead to depression, phobic avoidance, and persistent anxiety. (See *Panic disorder: Diagnostic criteria.*)

A first panic attack occurs unexpectedly. It doesn't immediately follow exposure to an anxiety-provoking situation. Later on, the patient may associate specific conditions, such as social pressure, heights, or crowds, with vulnerability to panic attack. Between attacks, the patient often worries whether he'll undergo another attack, and if so, when.

Rarely do these attacks occur only once. Patients frequently experience several attacks in the course of a week or even a day. The condition may pass after weeks or may last for years, with periods

Anxiety Disorders

Panic disorder: Diagnostic criteria

• The patient has experienced one or more unexpected panic attacks. True panic attacks do not occur immediately before or on exposure to a situation that usually causes anxiety. Nor are these attacks triggered by situations in which the person was the focus of others' attention.
• Either four attacks have occurred within a four-week period, or the patient has experienced at least a month of persistent fear of having another attack.
• At least four of the following symptoms developed during the attacks: chest pain or discomfort, choking, depersonalization or derealization, dizziness, unsteady feelings or faintness, dyspnea or smothering sensations, fear of dying, fear of going crazy or of doing something uncontrolled, hot flashes or chills, nausea or abdominal distress, numbness or paresthesias, palpitations or tachycardia, sweating, or trembling or shaking.
• Symptoms developed suddenly and increased in intensity within 10 minutes.
• An organic factor, such as amphetamine or caffeine intoxication or hyperthyroidism, didn't cause the attack.

of exacerbation and remission. Even during remissions, patients may endure limited symptom attacks, leaving them unable to leave home to perform routine activities.

Panic disorder usually doesn't begin until late adolescence or adult life, and often develops in response to a sudden loss. It may be triggered by severe separation anxiety experienced during early childhood. Recent evidence indicates biochemical functions of the brain may help to explain panic disorder. Certain individuals may be especially sensitive to chemicals in the body. When anxiety increases, this sensitivity intensifies. Complications of this disorder may include abuse of alcohol or anxiolytics. Most patients develop some symptoms of agoraphobia. (See *Agoraphobia,* page 38.)

Studies reveal increased risk of hypertension, peptic ulcer, and premature death from cardiac disease in patients with panic disorder. Mitral valve prolapse is 30% to 50% more frequent in patients with panic disorder than the general population. The relationship between the disorders remains obscure. A proposed genetic linkage is controversial.

Assessment. To assess a patient for panic disorder, obtain a thorough history and perform a physical examination.

Assess the patient for dyspnea or smothering sensations, choking, palpitations, or tachycardia. Does he feel dizzy, unsteady, or faint? Is he sweating, trembling, or shaking? Does he complain of nausea, abdominal distress, numbness, or paresthesias? Other symptoms may include diarrhea and hot flashes with sweating or chills.

Does the patient describe a sense of depersonalization or fear of losing control, going crazy, or dying? Does he seem preoccupied with feelings of terror, eeriness, and unreality, or display severely disrupted mental functioning? The patient may briefly experience delusional thinking, hallucinations, and a decreased ability to distinguish reality. Distorted perception may limit his ability to interact with the environment. Note, however, that some patients experience panic attacks without the characteristic sense of terror or other psychological symptoms.

Diagnosis. Panic and limited symptom attacks may be difficult to distinguish from a number of neurologic, cardiovascular, respiratory, or GI symptoms. Usually, the doctor will diagnose panic disorder only after ruling out possible organic causes, such as hypoglycemia, pheochromocytoma, and hyperthyroidism. Diagnosis is complicated because patients may fail to report the psychological symptoms of the attack.

Panic disorder frequently appears in patients with somatoform disorders (see Chapter 3). In fact, these patients are nearly 100 times more likely than the general population to have panic disorder. Their preoccupation with physical symptoms makes diagnosis of panic disorder difficult. They may also deny anxiety symptoms to avoid being stigmatized.

Psychoactive substance use or withdrawal may lead to symptoms of panic disorder. However, doctors will not diagnose panic disorder for attacks induced by ingesting a psychoactive substance.

Continued on page 38

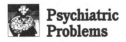
Anxiety Disorders

Agoraphobia

Agoraphobia refers to a fear of places or situations from which escape might be difficult or embarrassing, such as standing in a line or in a crowd, walking on a bridge, or traveling in a bus, train, or car.

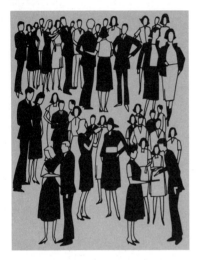

The patient with panic disorder may fear situations where help would be unavailable in the event of a panic attack. As a result, the person may refuse to travel alone and require a companion when away from home. Or he may tolerate intense anxiety during agoraphobic situations.

Usually the patient fears having a limited symptom attack: a single or small number of symptoms, such as dizziness or falling, depersonalization or derealization, loss of bladder or bowel control, vomiting, cardiac distress, cold clammy hands, dry mouth, dyspnea, faintness, increased pulse and blood pressure, palpitations, perspiration, and trembling.

In some cases, such symptoms have occurred in the past, and the patient may be preoccupied with fears of their recurrence. In other cases, the patient has never experienced any symptoms, but nevertheless fears that they may develop and be incapacitating or extremely embarrassing. In a few cases, the patient can't specify what symptoms he fears.

Agoraphobia most commonly begins when patients are in their twenties and thirties and may persist for years. Studies indicate that panic disorder without agoraphobia appears equally often in males and in females; panic disorder with agoraphobia occurs twice as often in females.

Other anxiety disorders—*continued*

Research indicates that one third of patients with panic disorder develop a secondary major depression, and about one fifth have had a major depressive disorder before developing panic disorder. If recurrent panic attacks occur during the course of a major depressive episode, the doctor will probably diagnose both a mood disorder and panic disorder. Similarly, if panic attacks recur during the course of somatoform disorder, the doctor will make an additional diagnosis of panic disorder.

The nervousness that most patients experience between attacks doesn't warrant diagnosis of generalized anxiety disorder. If the patient feels anxious for other reasons, the doctor may consider an additional diagnosis of generalized anxiety disorder.

A patient with a phobia may develop panic attack symptoms when exposed to the phobic stimulus. The attack occurs immediately before or upon exposure and decreases in intensity as the phobic stimulus withdraws. In panic disorder, however, even if the attacks are associated with agoraphobic situations, the patient never knows just when an attack will occur. Therefore, phobic episodes don't warrant a diagnosis of panic disorder, although phobia patients may have an unrelated panic disorder.

Intervention. Treatment may include behavioral therapy, supportive psychotherapy, or drug therapy, singly or in combination. Behavioral therapy works best when agoraphobia accompanies panic attack because identification of anxiety-inducing situations is easier. Psychotherapy may include cognitive techniques to help the patient assess the reality of his concerns and to view panic symptoms as a misinterpretation of essentially harmless physical sensations. (See *Relieving panic disorder.*)

Drug therapy. Drugs used to treat panic disorder include imipramine, phenelzine, and alprazolam. Like other tricyclic antidepressants (TCAs), *imipramine* has several drawbacks. Onset is delayed and adverse effects may include dry mouth, constipation, or orthostatic hypotension. In addition, during the early stages of therapy, patients may become worse. To minimize this affect, the doctor may initially order small doses (about 10 mg) and titrate upward according to the patient's response.

Monoamine oxidase (MAO) inhibitors are potentially useful against panic disorder. Doctors have used *phenelzine* to block attacks, relieve depression, and enhance confidence. Except for postural hypotension, MAO inhibitors don't induce most early TCA adverse effects. Unfortunately, as treatment proceeds, they may cause insomnia, weight gain, edema, nocturnal myoclonus, sexual dysfunction, and other untoward effects. Further, dietary precautions and the risk of hypertensive crises make many anxious patients uncomfortable.

Many patients can better tolerate *alprazolam.* This benzodiazepine acts quickly, is easy to administer, and is reasonably safe. Although the drug frequently provides dramatic results early on, it has a relatively short half-life and does have some drawbacks, such as possible abuse and dependency, rebound symptoms between doses, severe withdrawal symptoms, and early relapse.

Anxiety Disorders

Relieving panic disorder

Consider using the following nursing measures to help patients experiencing panic symptoms:
• If the patient experiences symptoms of fight or flight responses and feels out of control, remove him to a smaller, quieter space.
• Allow the patient to pace around the room (provided he isn't belligerent) to help expend energy.
• Stay with him if he needs physical restraint in order to feel safe.
• The patient's perceptual field may be narrowed, and excessive stimuli may cause him to feel overwhelmed. Dim bright lights or raise dim lights as necessary.
• Use statements such as "I know how you feel," "I won't let anything here hurt you," and "I'll stay with you" to assure the patient you are in control of the immediate situation. However, avoid using false reassurance.
• Once you've established rapport with the patient, you may touch him on his arm, shoulder, or hand. Without this rapport, however, it's better not to touch him. He may be too stimulated or frightened to find touch reassuring.
• Administer anxiolytics, as ordered.
• To understand the patient's perceptions and fears, encourage him to express his view of what is happening.
• To relieve tension, encourage the patient to cry.
• The patient may be so overwhelmed that he cannot follow lengthy or complicated processes. Speak in short, simple sentences, and slowly give one direction at a time. Avoid giving lengthy explanations and asking too many questions.

Because of these drawbacks, the doctor may initiate treatment with alprazolam and then add a TCA while tapering alprazolam. For patients who require a high-potency benzodiazepine but suffer rebound symptoms, clonazepam may prove effective.

Nearly twice as potent as alprazolam, *clonazepam* has a dosage range of 1 to 5 mg daily, divided in morning and bedtime doses. Sedation limits upward titration; give a low bedtime dose and titrate upward if symptoms persist and sedation lessens. If the patient doesn't readily adjust to sedation, give larger doses at bedtime than in the morning. Many patients, however, receive equal morning and bedtime doses without becoming sedated.

Within a few days, the drug should reduce panic attacks and overall anxiety. Some patients, however, develop depressive symptoms when started on clonazepam. If so, the doctor may order a TCA and withdraw clonazepam as patients respond to the TCA. If anxiety recurs despite antidepressant treatment, the doctor may return to combined drug therapy.

Phobic disorders

A phobia refers to an irrational, persistent fear of specific activities, objects, or situations that compels the patient to avoid the phobic stimulus. Although many people have irrational fears, such feelings usually do not interrupt daily living. Phobic anxiety, however, provokes behavior that disrupts work or social life.

Exposure to the phobic stimulus usually provokes an immediate response, with symptoms such as panic, diaphoresis, dyspnea, or tachycardia. The patient uses every available means to avoid the object of his dread. He realizes his terror is out of proportion to the threat posed by the object and is likely to seek help.

Most phobias begin early in life, when a child experiences separation anxiety and guilt about anger and sexuality. A deep inner threat provokes intense anxiety, which the patient projects onto some external object. The phobic object symbolizes the person's internal anxiety, although this connection may not always be obvious. Types of phobic disorders include social and simple phobia.

Social phobia describes an irrational fear of social scrutiny, humiliation, or embarrassment. The disorder often begins in late childhood or early adolescence and probably affects more males than females. Specific situations, such as urinating in a public lavatory or eating in company, may trigger a patient's fears. Other patients suffer a generalized form of social phobia stimulated by most social situations, such as fear of talking foolishly in front of others.

Typically, patients avoid threatening situations, but some force themselves to withstand the phobic situation and their consequent anxiety. Usually, the patient fears that others will sense his anxiety, creating a vicious cycle where anxiety further impairs social function, thus reinforcing the phobia.

The patient with social phobia may also have panic disorder or simple phobia. The disorder is usually chronic but rarely incapacitating. However, patients tend to abuse alcohol, barbiturates, and anxiolytics. Depression may set in if work or social life suffers.

Continued on page 40

Anxiety Disorders

Some simple phobias

Phobias abound. Here are the definitions of some simple ones:
● acrophobia—fear of heights
● agoraphobia—fear of open spaces
● algophobia—fear of pain
● astraphobia—fear of lightning
● claustrophobia—fear of closed spaces
● erythrophobia—fear of blushing
● hematophobia—fear of blood
● hydrophobia—fear of water
● iatrophobia—fear of doctors
● monophobia—fear of being alone
● mysophobia—fear of dirt and germs
● nyctophobia—fear of night and darkness
● pyrophobia—fear of fire
● senilophobia—fear of growing old
● sitophobia—fear of eating
● xenophobia—fear of strangers
● zoophobia—fear of animals.

Simple phobia describes the fear of situations or objects, other than social phobia or fear of panic attack. The most common simple phobias in the general population, though not necessarily among those seeking treatment, involve animals, particularly snakes, insects, dogs, and mice. Other common fears include witnessing blood or tissue injury (blood-injury phobia), closed spaces (claustrophobia), heights (acrophobia), and air travel (aviophobia).

As in social phobia, the person experiences marked anxiety just from anticipating an encounter with the phobic stimulus. Occasionally, he elects to endure the phobic situation and tolerate the consequent anxiety. Many people with blood-injury phobia experience vasovagal fainting if forced to witness an accident.

Anxiety decreases predictably when the phobic stimulus is withdrawn. Simple phobias rarely cause serious impairment unless the phobic object becomes difficult to avoid.

Simple phobias occur more often in females than in males. Animal phobias nearly always begin in childhood; blood-injury phobias most often appear in adolescence or early adulthood; and phobias of heights, air travel, driving, and closed spaces usually appear at about age 40 or later. Most simple childhood phobias disappear with treatment. However, adulthood phobias rarely abate without treatment. Simple phobia often coexists with social phobia and panic disorder.

Assessment. To assess the patient for social phobia, try to discover how strongly he feels about doing something embarrassing or humiliating in public. Ask the patient what situations make him anxious and what situations he chooses to avoid. Find out if he views his fear as excessive or unreasonable.

To assess for simple phobia, determine whether the patient has especially strong feelings toward any commonly feared objects or situations. (See *Some simple phobias.*)

Diagnosis. Avoiding social situations that commonly provoke uneasiness doesn't warrant a diagnosis of social phobia. Doctors will diagnose social phobia only if efforts to avoid the phobic stimulus interfere with the patient's career, daily life, or personal relationships, or if the phobia causes excessive distress.

In panic disorder with agoraphobia, the person may avoid social situations because he fears the embarrassment of having a panic attack, but this behavior doesn't warrant an additional diagnosis of social phobia. However, the patient may have an unrelated social phobia.

Intervention. Successful treatments for phobias include desensitization and reciprocal inhibition.

In *desensitization*, the therapist exposes the patient to a series of anxiety-provoking situations beginning with the least provocative one. Eventually, the provoking stimulus no longer causes anxiety.

Anxiety Disorders

Dealing with phobic behaviors

The following guidelines will help you to work with patients struggling with phobias:
• No matter how ridiculous the patient's phobia appears, do not trivialize it. To the patient, this behavior is a vital coping mechanism, needed to decrease or avoid anxiety. A facile pep talk or ridicule will only make the situation worse.
• The patient often perceives his phobic behavior as silly. Point out to the patient that his behavior serves as a way of coping with anxiety. You might say "You might think your behavior is silly, but it helps you feel better."
• Don't let the patient withdraw completely. If the patient is at home, help him take small steps to overcome fears by encouraging interaction with a supportive family member or friend.
• A gentle, supportive atmosphere will also help the patient remain involved with others. In social phobias, the patient fears criticism. Provide an accepting environment with positive reinforcement.
• Encourage the patient's participation in treatments such as desensitization therapy. However, do not force insight. Challenging the patient may aggravate anxiety or lead to panic.
• Provide for patient safety and comfort and monitor fluid and food intake, as needed. Certain phobias may inhibit food or fluid intake, disturb hygiene, and disrupt the patient's ability to rest.

In *reciprocal inhibition*, the therapist pairs the anxiety-provoking stimulus with a second stimulus that evokes a pleasant feeling strong enough to suppress the anxiety. The therapist may employ tranquilizers, biofeedback, meditation, or hypnosis.

Patients may also benefit from antidepressants coupled with supportive group therapy. Anxiety from simple phobia may require only occasional treatment with benzodiazepines. Beta blockers may help patients with social phobias.

Remember that forcing the patient to confront his phobia often compels him to panic or develop another phobia. Instead, help the patient to learn healthier ways of coping with anxiety. (See *Dealing with phobic behaviors.*)

Obsessive-compulsive disorder

Obsession refers to uncontrolled, recurrent thoughts, impulses, or images. Aware that the thoughts or impulses are intrusive and senseless, the patient tries to suppress them with other thoughts or activities.

The most common obsessions center on violence, contamination, and doubt. The patient may think about killing his brother, fear becoming infected by shaking hands, wonder about having hurt someone in a traffic accident that occurred years ago, or constantly anticipate a calamity. He may fear loss of control of behavior or bodily functions or think that his work is unacceptable to others.

The obsessive person is orderly, perfectionist, frugal, overly conscientious, and rigid, with high personal and moral standards and low tolerance for anxiety. He appears coherent and responds lucidly to a reality-test.

A patient may also express his anxiety through ritualistic symptoms, termed *compulsions*. Compulsive patients repeat bizarre and irrational activities according to a strict formula. Common compulsions include hand-washing, counting, cleaning, and touching. The patient may constantly check whether possessions are in their proper place and become anxious if things become disarranged. The patient feels compelled to act out the activity even against his desire to avoid it. Generally, he doesn't derive enjoyment from compulsive activity.

If the patient tries to resist performing his compulsive acts, his anxiety intensifies. Only yielding to the compulsion will relieve his tension. After repeated failure, the patient stops resisting. He may lose the desire to curb his behavior.

The compulsive person tends to exert tight control over his emotions, possibly leading to tense body posture, stubbornness, and flat affect. His life-style reflects a need for perfection and certainty.

Equally common in men and women, obsessive-compulsive disorder usually appears in adolescence or early adulthood, but sometimes begins in childhood. The disorder follows a chronic course with symptoms that periodically diminish and reappear. At worst, the patient may devote his life to acting out his compulsion. Compli-

Continued on page 42

Anxiety Disorders

What causes obsessive-compulsive disorder?

People once saw obsessive-compulsive behavior as a sign of demonic possession. Sigmund Freud among others recognized that obsessive-compulsive behavior enabled anxious individuals to cope. Sudden, bizarre thoughts served to distract the person's attention from other, possibly more upsetting, feelings.

Freud describes the disorder as a result of conflict between the ego and the id, in which impulses that are repugnant to the ego are controlled by denial, displacement, isolation, repression, reaction formation, suppression, and undoing. Research shows that obsessive-compulsive children are conformist, excessively mature, and try too hard to please adults.

Behaviorists see obsessive-compulsive disorder as a conditioned response to anxiety-provoking events. Associating anxiety with a neutral object or event causes obsessional preoccupation. Compulsive behavior is also learned. In the past, such behavior helped control the person's anxiety, so he practices it again, even though it's no longer helpful.

Other anxiety disorders—*continued*

cations include major depression and abuse of alcohol and anxiolytics.

Researchers disagree on the disorder's prevalence because many patients don't seek treatment until daily functioning becomes severely impaired. Mild forms of the disorder may occur fairly frequently. Some evidence indicates that obsessive-compulsive disorder occurs more often in close relatives of patients with Tourette's disorder. (See *What causes obsessive-compulsive disorder?*)

Be aware of the seriousness of obsessive-compulsive behaviors. Besides impairing a person's ability to function, they frequently threaten health and safety. For example, a person who compulsively washes his hands may contract severe infection because of breakdown of skin integrity. A mother obsessed with thoughts of killing her infant may neglect it completely rather than risk giving in to violent urges.

Assessment. When assessing obsessive-compulsive behavior, take note of themes that recur throughout the patient interview.

Because many patients recognize their thoughts and behavior as irrational and potentially harmful, they may seek psychiatric help. The patient may readily reveal obsessive thoughts because they are so disturbing. Questions such as "Do you think about this a lot?" or "How much trouble do these thoughts cause you?" may uncover still other obsessions.

Watch for symptoms of depression and anxiety. Determine if the patient avoids using public bathrooms or shaking hands with strangers. Also assess the patient's ability to meet his health and safety needs.

Diagnosis. Carried to excess, activities such as drinking, eating, or gambling may appear compulsive. But, unlike a true compulsion, the patient derives pleasure from indulgence and resists only out of fear of secondary consequences.

Nagging thoughts that recur as part of a major depressive episode do not constitute a true obsession because the patient doesn't perceive them as senseless. The depressed patient generally regards his ideas as meaningful, although possibly excessive. Obsessive thoughts may also form a secondary symptom of mood disorder or schizophrenia.

Distinguishing obsessive-compulsive disorder from schizophrenia. The thoughts that hound obsessive-compulsive patients may easily be confused with schizophrenic delusions. Usually, however, the obsessive-compulsive patient will at least consider the possibility that his belief is unfounded. Generally, you will not be able to cast doubt on a patient's irrational convictions if he has a delusion. Keep in mind, though, that some patients with obsessive-compulsive disorder may experience bizarre delusions and other symptoms that justify an additional diagnosis of schizophrenia.

Intervention. Supportive and insight-oriented psychotherapy may help the patient learn to control or eliminate his symptoms. Anti-

Anxiety Disorders

Coping with obsessive-compulsive behavior

Consider using the following nursing measures to help a patient with obsessive-compulsive disorder:
• Provide for basic needs such as rest, food, and grooming if the patient becomes so involved in ritualistic thoughts and behaviors that it causes self-neglect.
• Allow the patient ample time to perform ritualistic activity, within reasonable limits. The patient needs ritual defenses to reduce anxiety. Forcing the patient to give up these defenses will increase anxiety.
• To avoid increasing anxiety and causing greater need for compulsive behaviors, change the patient's environment as little as possible, and explain any necessary changes to him.
• Approach the patient in a caring way. Let him know you're aware of his behavior. For example, you might say "I noticed you've made your bed three times today; that must be very tiring for you." Help the patient explore feelings associated with the behavior. "What do you think about while you are performing your chores?"
• Help organize the patient's free time. Provide simple, structured tasks requiring concentration. To relieve the patient of decision-making anxieties and limit the time devoted to repetitive thinking, tell the patient what to do, rather than asking.
• Help the patient find alternative ways of controlling anxiety.
• Low self-esteem accompanies much ritualistic behavior. Reinforce the patient's self-esteem by demonstrating interest in his non-ritualistic behavior. For example, you might ask about a project he completed or a recent weekend trip.

depressants may be prescribed when depression accompanies the disorder. Researchers in the United States are studing clomipramine, a TCA available in some foreign countries that's thought to be more effective than current drug therapies.

The patient needs your warmth and support as well as time and patience. The patient's family and employer are probably frustrated by his behavior and may have insisted that he seek help. The patient may have lost his job and perceives entering treatment as an additional blow to his self-esteem. Caring for an ailing and demanding parent, divorce, or death of a loved one may also precipitate obsessive-compulsive behavior.

The patient's rigid thought patterns and strange behavior may make it difficult for you to relate to him. Endlessly repeated mannerisms can become frustrating. Instead of asking the patient to stop his behavior, try to accept it as an expression of his underlying conflicts and fears. Give him time to adopt healthier ways of coping. (See *Coping with obsessive-compulsive behavior.*)

Be alert for anger and frustration on your part regarding the patient's behavior. Seek consultation with a psychiatric liaison nurse or psychiatrist to help improve your coping methods.

Post-traumatic stress disorder
Unlike the anxiety disorders discussed earlier, post-traumatic stress disorder (PTSD) clearly and directly relates to traumatic events in the patient's past. Symptoms appear after a terrifying event outside the common scope of experience, such as:
• assault, burglary, rape, or torture
• military combat
• accidents, natural disasters, or acts of terrorism
• threat of death or severe injury
• fire or bombing
• witnessing of an assault on one's children, spouse, or close friends
• witnessing of a killing or serious injury, especially one involving family or friends
• sudden destruction of one's home or community.

Some experiences carry a higher risk of PTSD than others; for instance, a person is more likely to suffer PTSD after being tortured than after a car accident. Man-made calamities seem to induce more severe and long-lasting episodes of PTSD than natural disasters. (See *Post-traumatic stress disorder: Expressing the pain,* page 44.)

Afterward, the patient repeatedly relives the traumatic event. Usually, the patient has intrusive recollections or dreams. When reminded of the original event, the patient experiences intense stress and may display symptoms of anxiety. Holocaust survivors, for example, may tremble upon seeing an individual who reminds them of a uniformed guard, such as a firefighter or police officer. Rarely, the patient may enter dissociative states, lasting from a few seconds to several days, and act as though the event is still happening.

To minimize the pain of reliving the trauma, the patient avoids all stimuli associated with the event and may block out aspects of it

Continued on page 44

Anxiety Disorders

Post-traumatic stress disorder: Expressing the pain

A Vietnam veteran with post-traumatic stress disorder completed this drawing while undergoing art therapy, which focuses on self-expression through various forms of art. The dark figure in the foreground represents the veteran's conception of himself. His left hand holds a spear and is deliberately distorted. This distortion symbolizes the veteran's efforts to unite his prewar and postwar identities. The bartender, who observes him from the background, represents society.

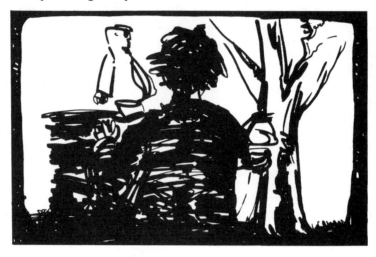

Other anxiety disorders—*continued*

from his memory. "Psychic numbing" or "emotional anesthesia" usually begins soon after the initial event. The patient may feel detached from others, stop responding to the outside world, lose interest in activities, or block emotions, especially those associated with intimacy, tenderness, and sexuality.

Assessment. Take a careful history. You'll be able to identify the external stressor that led to the patient's condition by carefully noting details given by him and his family. Keep in mind that the provoking event may have occurred as long as 6 months before symptoms appeared. You may find it hard to feel as strongly about the event as the patient does and may not appreciate the depth of his anguish. Be careful to avoid subtly trivializing the patient's pain, which could prevent him from sharing with you.

Note whether the patient startles easily; appears vigilant, tense, or excessively alert; or suffers from insomnia or memory defects. Ask the patient about guilt feelings. Many survivors of a catastrophe experience guilt because they lived while others died. Ask the patient what situations induce anxiety and if they remind him of the original trauma.

Ask the patient if he has difficulty in concentrating or in completing tasks. Note if he readily becomes irritable or fears losing control. In more severe forms of PTSD, patients may have unpredictable outbursts of aggressiveness or lose the ability to express angry feelings.

Assess for physical injury. The traumatic event may have led to malnutrition, head injury, or other damage. It may also cause panic.

Diagnosis. If symptoms last less than 1 month, the doctor will not diagnose PTSD. The doctor will diagnose the disorder as acute, if it lasts less than 6 months, or chronic, if it lasts more than 6 months. Depressive or organic mental disorder or another anxiety disorder may accompany PTSD.

Anxiety Disorders

Intervention. Behavioral therapy may help control the patient's panic. Crisis intervention focuses on the precipitating event and attempts to restore pre-crisis functioning as quickly as possible. The crisis therapist provides support while helping the patient relearn lost coping skills or develop new ones. The therapist may counsel individual patients, families, and groups. Group therapies work best if group members have all experienced similar trauma.

Antidepressant drugs, such as imipramine, may help reduce the incidence or severity of nightmares, flashbacks, panic, depression, insomnia, and other symptoms. Antipsychotic and antianxiety agents have proved less beneficial.

When in an emergency department or acute care setting, be especially alert for PTSD in rape or accident victims, and be prepared to direct the victim to the appropriate agency.

Anxiety in the hospitalized patient

In a medical hospital setting, you'll encounter many patients whose anxiety may not fit precisely into the definition of a recognized disorder but nevertheless requires serious consideration. Hospital patients routinely experience anxiety as a result of separation from friends and family, and from familiar surroundings. What's more, anxiety may appear as a major symptom of a medical condition.

Coping mechanisms
Most hospital patients employ various coping mechanisms to deal with stress, such as self-reassurance, denial, religious faith, and social support. Patients lacking support mechanisms, however, may yield to a sense of fear and vulnerability. Even well-adapted people may become anxious when facing a serious illness.

Many factors may contribute to failure to cope:
• a tendency to regress in the face of threat or, paradoxically, in a nurturing, passive setting
• sudden onset of a life-threatening disease
• lack of familial or other social support
• feelings of loneliness or abandonment
• unconscious guilt or anxiety associated with the illness or injury.

Unable to manage his anxiety, the patient becomes frightened, trembles, loses the ability to sleep, repeatedly seeks attention and reassurance, and complains of excessive pain and other symptoms. Children or the developmentally disabled are especially vulnerable to disabling anxiety. The anxious patient may disrupt procedures and interfere with your attempts to carry out your care plan. He may refuse to cooperate in treatment because he fears pain. He may disrupt your evaluation in an effort to minimize a serious condition.

Anxiety may also subvert rehabilitation. In a recent study of survivors of myocardial infarction, 80% of the patients who didn't return to work cited psychological impairment as the reason.

Treatment
Although hospitalization may worsen a patient's anxiety, it may also offer him the first opportunity to relieve it. The patient may benefit from evaluation by a psychiatric liaison nurse (PLN). A specialist in the field of psychiatric nursing, the PLN is charged with making sure patients receiving medical treatment are able to obtain needed emotional care. She may be employed in a medical-surgical ward, intensive or coronary care unit, emergency department, neurologic or other speciality unit, hospice center, nursing home, rehabilitation center, or other long-term care facility. As a member of the treatment team, the PLN may:
• assess patients for depression, delayed bereavement reactions, suicide risk, potential for violence, involvement in family conflict, and other signs of distress. This assessment may include the use of advanced diagnostic methods.
• evaluate patients who are withdrawn, manipulative, domineering, confused, angry, threatening, or uncooperative.

After evaluation by a PLN, the patient often may receive psychotherapy, group support, instruction on stress management techniques, or anxiolytic or antidepressant drug therapy. Supportive or insight-oriented psychotherapy may help him, though limits on time may deny him the advantages of long-term therapy. Behavioral and cognitive techniques may help the patient whose condition is complicated by generalized anxiety, phobias, or panic disorder symptoms.

Anxiety-related Disorders: The Mind-Body Connection

Barbara Gross Braverman, a psychotherapist in private practice in Philadelphia, Pa., wrote this chapter. She earned her BSN from Temple University in Philadelphia and her MSN from Wayne State University in Detroit, Mich.

In any clinical setting, you're likely to encounter patients with anxiety so overpowering it produces physical symptoms. Such patients may experience memory lapses, lose touch with reality, seek treatment for pain that has no organic cause, feign insanity, or inflict injury on themselves. Some develop multiple personalities.

Because anxiety-related disorders mimic organic diseases, they're frequently misdiagnosed. Even when they're detected, they prove difficult to treat. That's because patients derive psychological benefits from their symptoms and are likely to resist change.

This chapter will prepare you for the challenge of caring for patients with such anxiety-related conditions as dissociative, somatoform, and factitious disorders.

Dissociative disorders

Dissociation refers to an unconscious defense mechanism that keeps troubling thoughts out of a patient's awareness. In this disorder, the patient experiences sudden, temporary changes in consciousness, identity, and motor function. His behaviors represent an escape from feelings that threaten his sense of self. The patient may:
- forget stressful experiences
- lose touch with reality
- forget who he is and assume a new identity
- wander aimlessly, ending up in a new city.

A dissociative disorder may originate from some deeply stressful event, such as physical or sexual abuse, death of a loved one, combat, or natural disaster. The revised third edition of the *Diagnostic and Statistical Manual of Mental Disorders* (DSM-III-R) identifies five types of dissociative disorders:
- psychogenic amnesia
- psychogenic fugue
- multiple personality disorder
- depersonalization disorder
- unspecified dissociative disorder.

Once classified as a dissociative disorder, sleepwalking (somnambulism) now falls under the heading of sleep disorders.

Psychogenic amnesia. The most common dissociative disorder, psychogenic amnesia renders patients unable to remember events that occurred during a well-defined time period. Too all-encompassing to dismiss as mere forgetfulness, psychogenic amnesia can't be traced to an organic mental disorder or alcohol or drug use. Four main types have been identified. (See *Understanding psychogenic amnesia.*)

Symptoms usually follow a deeply stressful event, such as engaging in an extramarital love affair, losing one's livelihood, disobeying a strict parent, or violating a long-held religious belief. Psychogenic amnesia may also result from an accident, assault, or other threat of injury or death. Except in wartime, this disorder most commonly

Anxiety-related Disorders

Understanding psychogenic amnesia

Type	Example
Localized or circumscribed Patient can't recall anything that occurred for several hours or days after a traumatic event. Most common type of psychogenic amnesia.	Woman survives assault and rape but can't remember what happened for several days afterward.
Selective Patient loses recall of only certain parts of a traumatic event. Less common than localized amnesia.	Wife can recall making funeral arrangements after her husband's death but can't remember who attended the funeral.
Generalized Patient loses recall of all events in his life. Less common than localized and selective amnesia.	Soldier returning from war can't remember who he is or where he's from.
Continuous Patient loses his memory beginning with a traumatic event and continuing up to the present.	Teenager can't remember anything since a homosexual encounter the month before.

afflicts adolescents and young women. The degree of functional impairment experienced during the amnestic period varies according to the severity of precipitating events. Most patients recover quickly.

Psychogenic fugue. During a psychogenic fugue, the patient forgets his identity, abandons familiar surroundings, and travels aimlessly. He may take on a new name and identity and, possibly, commit violent or criminal acts. Fugues usually last only a few hours or a few days. Occasionally, however, they may persist for months and may lead the patient thousands of miles away from home.

Like psychogenic amnesia, psychogenic fugue also occurs after episodes of severe psychological stress, such as rejection by a loved one, family argument, military conflict, or natural disaster. Fugues do not originate in organic problems or drug use. Heavy alcohol use, however, can predispose a patient to the disorder.

Typically, the patient recovers rapidly and rarely experiences relapses. However, he usually doesn't remember what happened during the fugue.

Multiple personality disorder. Once considered rare, multiple personality disorder is now recognized as a more common malady. In this disorder, patients have two or more well-defined personalities or personality states. *Personality* describes a relatively consistent pattern of behavior and attitudes, revealed in a wide variety of social and personal situations. *Personality state* describes a pattern of behavior and attitudes expressed in a more limited context.

Because multiple personality disorder involves disturbances of memory and identity, doctors frequently mistake it for a variety of psychological and organic disorders. The personality that goes for treatment often knows little or nothing about the other personalities, making diagnosis even more complicated. Nevertheless, affected patients do share some common characteristics:
• The patient's behavior will fall under the control of at least 2 distinct personalities at different times. With most patients, fewer

Continued on page 48

Anxiety-related Disorders

Dissociative disorders—*continued*

than 10 personalities will ever appear, though as many as 100 personalities are possible.
• The transition from one personality to another usually will occur in seconds or minutes, though it may take hours or days.
• An interview conducted with the patient under sedation or hypnosis may provoke takeover by a new personality.
• The patient likely suffered sexual abuse during childhood.
• The condition is chronic, although the frequency of switching between personalities may decrease with age.
• The patient usually seeks help during adulthood.
• When other personalities take over, the patient may experience episodes of amnesia or memory distortion.
• Patient history may reveal attempts at suicide or self-mutilation, violent activity, or dependence on drugs or alcohol.
• The patient is three to nine times more likely to be female than male and has a greater than average likelihood of a family history of the disorder.

The different personalities. The disorder's severity varies according to the nature of the personalities, their relationship, and to a lesser extent, their number. Personalities might be exact opposites in attitude, behavior, and self-image. For example, a quiet, shy bachelor might alternate with an outgoing, promiscuous playboy. Personalities might distinguish themselves in how they respond to problems. A patient may have one personality that responds to aggression by running away, a second masochistic personality that willingly submits to aggression, and a third that fights back. One personality might hold down a job and function independently, while another might be dysfunctional. Studies have shown that separate personalities in the same patient can even have different physiologic characteristics, such as different eyeglass prescriptions or different responses to the same medication. These personalities may respond differently to psychological tests and have different IQs. In addition, some personalities might report that they're of the opposite sex, a different age or race, or from a different family than other personalities, and behave accordingly. During the course of a patient's life, the proportion of time that each personality controls will vary.

Personalities of the same age often occur in groups of two or more, with one personality acting as the protector of the others. Most personalities have names, often with symbolic meaning. A personality that likes music may ask to be called "Melody." Occasionally, a personality's name may reveal its relationship to other personalities, for example, "the Protector."

Psychosocial stress or environmental or social cues with special meaning for the patient may prompt takeover by a new personality. Conflicts or agreements among co-personalities may precipitate this change. While the patient who comes in for treatment understands little if anything about his condition, his multiple personalities are well acquainted with each other. When a new personality takes control, other personalities might eavesdrop or influence what's happening. Personalities might report listening to other personalities, talking to them, or participating together in activities. On the

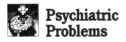

Anxiety-related Disorders

Why depersonalization develops

Researchers have attributed the development of depersonalization disorder to both biological and psychological causes.

Organic theory
Depersonalization stems from a physical problem, perhaps an abnormality in a specific area of the brain (as occurs in a temporal lobe seizure).

General psychiatric theory
Depersonalization stems from anxiety, dysphoric affect, and disorganized thinking.

Psychoanalytic theory
Depersonalization stems from the struggle between conflicting identities and self-images. When a toddler realizes he's separate from his mother, he also starts to imitate and identify with his parents (called separation-individuation). But if a young child has no suitable parent to identify with, his self-image will be weak, leading to depersonalization. In adulthood, if faced with a loss, he regresses to avoid anxiety, at the same time watching himself as if from the outside.

other hand, some personalities might be aware of other ones but not interact with them.

Some patients may deny episodes of amnesia or time and memory distortions, fearing accusations of lying or insanity. Other patients, however, won't even realize they've lost hours or days, because one dominant personality either fabricates memories or has access to the memories of the others and uses them to cover periods of amnesia.

Often, alternate personalities exhibit symptoms, such as mood changes or anxiety, indicating a coexisting mental problem. But whether these symptoms denote coexisting disorders or just associated features of multiple personality remains unclear.

Depersonalization disorder. Depersonalization describes a deep feeling of unreality and detachment from the environment. The patient walks in a dreamlike, numbed state and views himself from a distance, as if watching a mechanical doll. No longer does he feel in control of his behavior or speech. Objects become distorted in size and shape. The patient is aware of and disturbed by these unnatural sensations.

The patient usually doesn't seek help but is referred by others. Doctors diagnose depersonalization disorder (also called depersonalization neurosis) when the condition interferes with occupational or social functioning.

One theory suggests that depersonalization develops when a person with low self-esteem obsessively scrutinizes himself. An introspective person with unrealistically high standards of behavior is especially vulnerable. Such a patient tends to focus on his insecurities, thereby aggravating feelings of failure. Eventually, anxiety and depression become so intense that the patient becomes detached from himself and his surroundings. (See *Why depersonalization develops.*)

Episodes range from mild to severe, depending partly on associated conditions such as anxiety or fear of insanity. Single, brief episodes of depersonalization may occur in as many as 70% of young adults. The prevalence of persistent or recurrent episodes is unknown.

Predisposing factors include fatigue, physical pain, such altered states of consciousness as hypnosis or meditation, anxiety, depression, severe stress, or trauma such as a car crash or military combat. Other characteristics of depersonalization disorder include:
• onset in adolescence or early adulthood. The disorder rarely develops after age 40.
• chronic recurrence, with episodes appearing suddenly and disappearing gradually, and periods of remission. Exacerbations usually result from mild anxiety or depression.
• concurrent hypochondriasis or drug or alcohol addiction.

Unspecified dissociative disorder. Occasionally, a patient will present symptoms that suggest a dissociative disorder but don't quite fit into any category. Examples include trancelike states resulting from brainwashing or terrorist indoctrination or detachment from reality without the other signs of depersonalization.

Continued on page 50

Anxiety-related Disorders

Dissociative disorders—*continued*

Assessment

When assessing for a dissociative disorder, remember that many other emotional disorders and some organic illnesses have similar symptoms. To lay the groundwork for the doctor's diagnosis, consider each symptom carefully. The patient may require a physical assessment to rule out an organic cause. (See *Differential diagnosis: Dissociative disorders.*)

Consider the patient's personality type and any signs of changed behavior. Begin by asking if he's recently experienced a crisis or stressful event, and ask him to describe it.

Other questions you might ask the patient include:
• Have you experienced sleepwalking, trancelike states, memory loss, vivid dreams, or fainting spells?
• Do you feel a sense of unreality or detachment from your surroundings?
• Have you ever felt you were outside your body, as if observing yourself?

Observe the patient for changes in his state of awareness, level of consciousness, and eye or facial expression. Note whether he seems not quite with you in thought and feeling. In addition, look for characteristic behaviors associated with each of the five types of dissociative disorders.

Planning

When writing your nursing care plan, focus on helping the patient to identify conflicts or sources of stress, regain his sense of self, and find effective ways to cope with his anxiety. Before determining your care plan, develop the nursing diagnoses by identifying the patient's actual or potential problem, then relating it to its cause. Possible nursing diagnoses for a patient with a dissociative disorder include the following:
• anxiety; related to dissociative disorder
• coping, ineffective individual; related to dissociative disorder
• thought process, altered (memory loss); related to psychogenic amnesia or multiple personality disorder
• violence, potential for; related to psychogenic fugue
• grieving, dysfunctional; related to sudden loss of spouse
• sensory-perceptual alteration; related to dissociative disorder
• self-concept, disturbance in; related to dissociative disorder
• self-concept, disturbance in; related to personal identity.

The sample nursing care plan on page 52 shows expected outcomes, nursing interventions, and discharge planning for one of the nursing diagnoses listed above. However, you'll want to individualize your care plan to fit the needs of your patient.

Intervention

After an episode of psychogenic amnesia or psychogenic fugue, organic illness such as temporal lobe epilepsy must first be ruled out. Once this is done, supportive psychotherapy can help identify the conflict or threat behind the patient's anxiety. Therapy provides insight into the patient's thoughts, feelings, and behavior, and helps him establish and maintain interpersonal relationships and deal

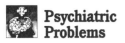
Anxiety-related Disorders

more effectively with anxiety. Under psychotherapy, most of these patients make steady progress.

Expect to encounter much greater difficulty when treating multiple personality disorder. Affected patients usually need intense, long-term psychotherapy, perhaps including hypnosis or art, music, or

Continued on page 52

Differential diagnosis: Dissociative disorders

Because many organic and psychological disorders can closely resemble dissociative disorders, evaluating the patient's symptoms requires careful attention.

Identifying psychogenic amnesia

Use the following guidelines to distinguish psychogenic amnesia from organic and other disorders:

Organic mental disorder. Unlike psychogenic amnesia, memory disturbances that occur as part of an organic mental disorder aren't stress-related, and recent memory is usually more impaired than remote memory. Full return of memory is rare; if memory returns, it usually does so gradually. Problems with attention span and affect may also occur.

Psychoactive substance–induced intoxication. Patients experience blackouts and can't recall events that occurred during the intoxication. Substance abuse and incomplete memory return distinguish this condition from psychogenic amnesia.

Alcohol amnestic disorder. The patient loses short-term memory, an impairment not seen in psychogenic amnesia. Other characteristics include blunted affect, confabulation, and lack of awareness of the memory impairment.

Postconcussion amnesia. Patients often can't remember what happened just before the trauma; in psychogenic amnesia, patients usually can't remember what happened afterward. Hypnosis or amobarbital interview can help distinguish postconcussion amnesia from psychogenic amnesia. Prompt recovery of lost memory also indicates a psychogenic cause for the amnesia.

Seizures. Memory loss caused by seizures occurs suddenly, accompanied by motor abnormalities. Repeated EEGs usually reveal abnormalities not present in psychogenic amnesia. During the postictal state, patients recover gradually.

Catatonic stupor. Patients may experience mutism but usually don't suffer memory loss. Other characteristics include rigidity, posturing, and negativism.

Malingering. Patients simulate amnesia, making diagnosis difficult. Hypnosis and amobarbital interview may help rule out psychogenic amnesia, though some patients will continue to malinger in a trancelike state.

Recognizing psychogenic fugue

Use the following guidelines to distinguish psychogenic fugue from multiple personality and other disorders:

Multiple personality disorder. Memory distortions may cause fugue symptoms, but unlike psychogenic fugue, the disorder isn't limited to a single episode. Fugue patients also don't shift identities over and over. Another difference: patients with multiple personality disorders have identity distur-

bances during childhood, whereas patients with psychogenic fugue don't encounter such problems until the fugue's onset.

Psychogenic amnesia. Like psychogenic fugue, patients suddenly can't recall important events or remember who they are. However, they don't travel or assume new identities.

Temporal lobe seizures. Patients are dysphoric and don't assume new identities. Usually, psychosocial stress doesn't precipitate their state.

Malingering. Patients pretend they can't recall their identity as well as simulate amnesia, making diagnosis difficult. Hypnosis and amobarbital interview can help rule out psychogenic fugue.

Identifying multiple personality disorder

Be careful not to confuse multiple personality disorder with psychogenic fugue or other conditions:

Psychogenic fugue and psychogenic amnesia. These disorders may resemble multiple personality disorder, but patients don't experience repeated identity shifts and usually endure amnesia or fugue for only one brief episode.

Schizophrenia and mood disorder with psychotic features. These disorders can be confused with multiple personality disorder because the patient may also report being controlled or influenced by others and hearing or talking with voices.

Complaints of being possessed. This may occur as a symptom of multiple personality disorder (the patient interprets takeover by an alternate personality as possession) or a psychotic delusion.

Borderline personality disorder. Doctors sometimes mistake the appearance of new personalities for instability in mood, self-image, or interpersonal behavior, which are common signs of borderline personality disorder. In addition, patients may suffer concurrent mental disorders that obscure the presence of multiple personality disorder.

Malingering. Differentiating between multiple personality disorder and malingering may require obtaining additional information from hospital and police records, family members, employers, and friends.

Pinpointing depersonalization disorder

Symptoms of depersonalization may occur in schizophrenia, mood disorders, organic mental disorders (especially intoxication and withdrawal), other anxiety disorders, personality disorders, and seizures. However, doctors do not diagnose depersonalization disorder unless symptoms affect the person's social or occupational life.

Anxiety-related Disorders

Sample nursing care plan: Dissociative disorder

Nursing diagnosis	Expected outcomes
Self-concept, disturbance in; related to dissociative disorder	The patient will: • express feelings of greater control over his actions. • indicate that he has become less detached from his environment. • demonstrate improved social and occupational functioning.
Nursing interventions • Provide a safe environment. • Refer the patient to a therapist. • Give feedback to the patient about his behavior. • Support the patient, demonstrate personal acceptance, and stay involved in his care. • Praise the patient's efforts and accomplishments as he learns to cope with stress.	**Discharge planning** • Typically, doctors do not order hospitalization for dissociative patients. However, if for some reason the patient is hospitalized, provide follow-up care as necessary.

Dissociative disorders—*continued*

dance therapy. During a crisis, the doctor may order hospitalization in a psychiatric facility. Although the disorder's chief symptoms don't respond to medication, the doctor may order antidepressants, anxiolytics, and sedatives to treat anxiety and depression. (See *Pathway to treating multiple personality disorder.*) Alcohol and drug abuse, if present, must also be treated.

In depersonalization disorders, psychotherapy attempts to improve self-esteem. Help the patient avoid excessive introspection by teaching him how to replace negative thoughts with positive ones. Drug therapy appears to be ineffective; phenothiazines actually intensify feelings of depersonalization. Expect improvement to take considerable time, and watch for symptoms to worsen in times of stress.

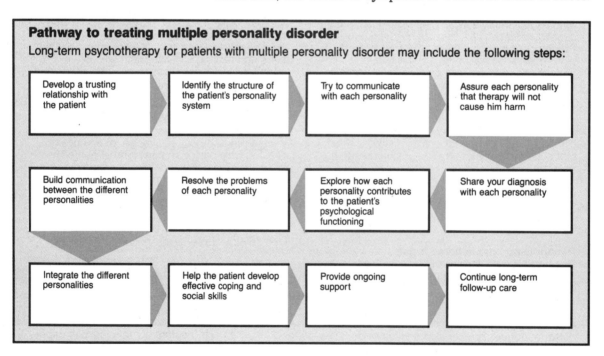

Pathway to treating multiple personality disorder

Long-term psychotherapy for patients with multiple personality disorder may include the following steps:

Develop a trusting relationship with the patient → Identify the structure of the patient's personality system → Try to communicate with each personality → Assure each personality that therapy will not cause him harm

Build communication between the different personalities → Resolve the problems of each personality → Explore how each personality contributes to the patient's psychological functioning → Share your diagnosis with each personality

Integrate the different personalities → Help the patient develop effective coping and social skills → Provide ongoing support → Continue long-term follow-up care

Anxiety-related Disorders

Tips for treating dissociative disorders

• Relate to all aspects of the patient's personality—don't just focus on his symptoms.
• Encourage staff members to be consistent in how they approach the patient and to set reasonable limits on behavior.
• Help relieve the patient's anxiety and meet his dependency needs by providing a safe, protected environment, but don't let him manipulate you into doing what he can do himself.
• Uncover the patient's basic problems and conflicts by learning his life story, his defense mechanisms, and the stressful event that precipitated the symptom.
• Build a relationship of trust, security, teaching, and support that encourages the patient to vent his feelings.
• Expect the patient to test your trustworthiness and patience.
• Help foster greater self-esteem as the patient struggles toward maturity and stability.
• Help the patient learn to relate to others by encouraging him to control his impulses, to think before acting, and to develop problem-solving skills.
• Encourage the patient to develop new interests, long-term goals, and strategies for coping with stress and anxiety.
• Explore your own feelings of anger and frustration. You may have to consult with a psychiatric liaison nurse for help.

Nursing interventions focus on supporting the patient and helping him learn to cope with anxiety. (See *Tips for treating dissociative disorders*.)

Evaluation

Base your evaluation on the patient's expected outcomes listed in the nursing care plan. To determine if the patient's improved, ask yourself the following questions:
• Does the patient state that he feels more in control of his behavior?
• Does he say that he feels like a participant in rather than an observer of his environment?
• Is he functioning better at work and in social situations?

The answers to these and similar questions will help you evaluate your patient's status and the effectiveness of your care plan. Keep in mind that these questions stem from the sample nursing care plan. Your questions may differ.

Other anxiety-related disorders

Somatoform disorders

The patient with a somatoform disorder complains of physical symptoms and typically travels from doctor to doctor in search of sympathetic and enthusiastic treatment. Physical examinations and laboratory tests, however, fail to uncover an organic basis for these symptoms. Because the patient doesn't produce the symptoms intentionally or feel a sense of control over them, he's usually unable to accept that his illness has a psychological cause.

Two current theories, the psychodynamic model and the behavioral model, help explain the origin of somatoform disorders. According to the *psychodynamic model*, symptoms express an underlying conflict. For example, hypochondriasis may provide an outlet for a person who wants to express dependency and anger without losing self-esteem or being blamed by others. According to the *behavioral model*, psychosomatic symptoms result from learned behavior. The patient desires a secondary gain such as more attention, less responsibility, or higher family status. After being ill, the patient realizes that having physical symptoms satisfies part of his needs. The response his illness elicits from others reinforces this learned behavior.

This section discusses six types of somatoform disorders:
• body dysmorphic disorder
• conversion disorder
• hypochondriasis
• somatization disorder
• somatoform pain disorder
• undifferentiated somatoform disorder.

Body dysmorphic disorder. Previously called dysmorphophobia, body dysmorphic disorder refers to a preoccupation with an imaginary defect in appearance. Complaints usually focus on facial features: wrinkles, spots on the skin, excessive hair, facial swelling, or the

Continued on page 54

Anxiety-related Disorders

Other anxiety-related disorders—*continued*

shape of the nose, mouth, jaw, or eyebrows. Less frequently, complaints center on the feet, hands, breasts, back, or other parts of the body. Patients sometimes have minor physical irregularities, hardly sufficient to warrant their excessive concern. This disorder may be more common than previously thought. It usually develops during adolesence or the twenties, lasts for several years, and accompanies concurrent depressive syndrome and obsessive-compulsive personality traits.

Patients visit plastic surgeons or dermatologists repeatedly, trying to correct the imagined body defect. Unnecessary surgical procedures may follow. The imagined defect may stop patients from working or going out socially.

Conversion disorder. Previously called hysteria, hysterical neurosis, or conversion reaction, conversion disorder involves a change in or loss of physical functioning stemming from a psychological conflict or need. Less common now than in the past, you're most likely to care for conversion disorder patients if you work in an orthopedic or neurologic unit or in a military setting (especially during wartime).

According to the psychodynamic model, the patient may develop conversion disorder to block out an internal conflict. For example, during an argument, a patient with difficulty expressing anger might develop aphonia. If a wife sees her husband involved with another woman, she may express her conflict over confronting it by developing blindness. The symptom acquires a symbolic value that represents and partly solves the underlying psychological conflict.

The behavioral model holds that the patient seeks a secondary gain, such as avoiding a particular activity or obtaining emotional support. For example, a soldier may suddenly develop a paralyzed hand to avoid firing his gun. A man who's afraid his wife will run off might suddenly be unable to walk or stand, even though he can move his legs normally.

Symptoms such as paralysis, aphonia, seizures, blindness, tunnel vision, anosmia, or anesthesia may mimic a neurologic disorder. Globus hystericus, the sensation of a lump in the the throat, probably occurs most often in women. When the endocrine and autonomic nervous system are involved, vomiting or pseudocyesis may occur. Most patients experience one symptom per incident. This symptom will usually be serious enough to interrupt the patient's daily activities. It lasts for a short time, beginning and ending abruptly. If subsequent episodes occur, symptoms may vary in site and nature. Recurrent symptoms may indicate a chronic condition.

Other characteristic features in conversion disorder patients include:
• onset during adolescence or early adulthood (though the disorder may appear during middle age or later)
• exposure to others with real or conversion symptoms, severe psychosocial stress, and coexisting physical disorders that provide a prototype for the symptoms (see *Distinguishing conversion disorder seizures from organic seizures*)

Anxiety-related Disorders

Distinguishing conversion disorder seizures from organic seizures

Signs and symptoms	Organic seizure	Conversion disorder seizure
Full loss of consciousness	yes	no
Seizures occur when alone	yes	no
Loss of pupillary and deep reflexes	yes	no
Tongue biting	yes	no
Incontinence	yes	no
Cyanosis or pallor	yes	no
Facial flushing	no	yes
Resistance to efforts by others to open eyes	no	yes
Withdrawal of head upon feeling supraorbital pressure	no	yes

• disuse atrophy or contractures that can to lead to a loss of function or disfigurement
• disfigurement or incapacity from unnecessary medical procedures or surgery
• *la belle indifférence*, an indifferent attitude toward the impairment (also present in some seriously ill medical patients).

Hypochondriasis. The patient with this disorder harbors an unrealistic fear of developing a serious disease. Physical assessment shows no serious organic problems, but that does not reassure the patient. Instead, he responds with anger, frustration, and disappointment.

Preoccupied with normal body functions, such as heartbeat, sweating, or peristalsis, or with minor physical problems, such as a small sore or an occasional cough, the patient readily interprets almost anything as evidence of a serious disease. He may fear disease in several body systems or may focus in a specific organ, such as the heart (cardiac neurosis).

Equally common in males and females, the disorder usually first appears between age 20 and 30. The obsession with body functions often interferes with job performance and family or social life. In severe cases, the person actually becomes a bedridden invalid. However, many hypochondriasis patients do recover.

When a medical visit fails to elicit a diagnosis, the patient will "doctor-shop," creating frustration and anger on the part of the patient and doctor alike. Ironically, doctors may fail to discover real physical disorders because the patient's imaginary symptoms obscure everything else.

Look for the following characteristics in patients with hypochondriasis:
• a personal or family history of organic disease
• recent severe psychosocial stress
• a history of repeated diagnostic procedures, such as exploratory surgery
• chronic complaints, with symptoms more unbearable during some periods than others.

Somatization disorder. Patients with somatization disorder (once called hysteria or Briquet's syndrome) experience repeated, multiple

Continued on page 56

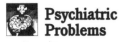

Anxiety-related Disorders

Symptoms of somatization disorder

Cardiopulmonary symptoms
• shortness of breath (without exertion)
• palpitations
• chest pain
• dizziness

GI symptoms
• abdominal pain (excluding menstruation)
• nausea and vomiting (excluding motion sickness)
• flatulence
• diarrhea
• intolerance to foods

Female reproductive symptoms
• irregular menses
• excessive menstrual bleeding
• vomiting throughout pregnancy

Pseudoneurologic symptoms
• amnesia
• dysphagia
• loss of voice or hearing
• double or blurred vision
• blindness
• fainting or loss of consciousness
• seizures
• difficulty walking, weakness, or paralysis
• urinary retention or dysuria

Pain
• in extremities
• in back
• during urination

Sexual symptoms
• burning sensation in sexual organs or rectum (except during intercourse)
• sexual indifference
• dyspareunia or lack of pleasure during sex
• impotence

Other anxiety-related disorders—*continued*

somatic complaints with no discernible physical cause. Most complaints fall into one of the following categories:
• conversion or pseudoneurologic symptoms (paralysis, blindness)
• chest, abdominal, or lower back pain
• gynecologic symptoms (dysmenorrhea)
• psychosexual symptoms (sexual apathy).

As early as preadolescence, the patient, usually female, displays a variety of physical symptoms, such as seizures, depression, headache, and abdominal pain. Usually, symptoms first appear during the teens. Rarely, onset may occur in the twenties. As the disorder progresses, the patient develops chronic, fluctuating complaints and frequently seeks medical attention, often from a variety of doctors. (See *Symptoms of somatization disorder.*) This may lead to unnecessary procedures and abuse of medications.

The patient's history is complex and confused. The patient who seeks psychological help does so because of severe, sometimes incapacitating depression. The patient also experiences job, marriage, and interpersonal problems and frequently threatens or attempts suicide. What's more, the patient may have auditory hallucinations—most frequently hearing her name called. Histrionic personality disorder and, rarely, antisocial personality disorder may also be present.

Both biological and environmental factors contribute to development of this disorder. 10% to 20% of women whose close biological relatives have somatization disorder develop the condition. Men related to women with this disorder face an increased risk of antisocial personality disorder or drug or alcohol abuse. Studies show that adoptive parents with somatization disorder increase their children's risk of developing antisocial personality disorder, drug or alcohol addiction, and somatization disorder. This disorder rarely disappears spontaneously.

Somatoform pain disorder. A preoccupation with pain dominates the lives of patients with this disorder. Patients may experience symptoms that mimic organic diseases, such as angina or sciatica, as well as sensory or motor changes, such as paresthesias or muscle spasm. No pathologic mechanism accounts for the pain.

Like patients with other somatoform disorders, these patients frequently doctor-shop. Most patients are female. Many of them begin working at a very young age, hold physically taxing or overly routine jobs, and become workaholics. About half experience physical trauma immediately before the onset of pain.

While onset may occur from childhood to old age, the patient usually first experiences symptoms during her thirties or forties. The attack is sudden and increases in intensity over weeks or months. Most patients tolerate their symptoms for several years before seeking help.

In some cases, a clear relationship exits between a psychological conflict and the beginning or exacerbation of pain. Sometimes the pain is symbolic. For example, a patient whose father died of heart

Anxiety-related Disorders

Assessing somatoform disorders

Use the following questions as guidelines when evaluating a patient for a possible somatoform disorder:
- ☐ Do the symptoms together with clinical findings point to a diagnosis of somatoform disorder?
- ☐ Did the patient experience major emotional stress before the symptoms started? Does elimination of stress relieve the symptoms?
- ☐ Do the patient's symptoms fit a known pattern of organic illness, or are they more obscure?
- ☐ Do the patient's emotional conflicts provide an explanation of his symptoms?
- ☐ Do the symptoms have an unusual psychological significance for the patient?
- ☐ Does the patient achieve secondary gains from the symptoms?
- ☐ Do the symptoms justify a psychiatric diagnosis?

disease might have pain mimicking angina. The pain often allows the patient to avoid unpleasant activities or to obtain needed emotional support. In other cases, no evidence of psychological etiology exists.

Patients with somatoform pain disorder may exhibit the following characteristics:
- symptoms of conversion disorder or depression, especially anhedonia and insomnia
- use of minor tranquilizers and narcotics, without relief
- repeated, unnecessary surgery
- incapacitation and inability to work
- assumption of an invalid role.

Evidence suggests that close biological relatives of people with this disorder have a high incidence of painful injuries, illnesses, depression, and alcohol dependence.

Undifferentiated somatoform disorder. Most patients who develop physical complaints with no known organic cause will not meet the full criteria for a somatization disorder. They might have one symptom, such as difficulty swallowing, or many symptoms, such as anorexia, fatigue, and GI problems. These patients are as likely to be men as women, and frequently experience anxiety and depression. The condition may recur or disappear after a single episode. The patient's overall functioning usually suffers less than in somatization disorder.

Doctors will not diagnose undifferentiated somatoform disorder if the symptoms last less than 6 months or if they coincide with another somatoform disorder, a sexual pain disorder, or a mood, anxiety, sleep, or psychotic disorder.

Assessment. Because somatoform disorders can mimic organic ones, diagnosis is complicated. Many doctors mistakenly send patients for multiple tests, procedures, and even operations. You may assist in assigning a proper diagnosis by thoroughly reviewing both physiologic and psychological data. (See *Assessing somatoform disorders.*) You may want to ask such questions as:
- When did your symptoms first appear?
- Have you been feeling anxious or depressed?
- What medical treatment have you received in the past?

When assessing for *body dysmorphic disorder*, discuss the patient's concerns about his appearance and assess whether these concerns are excessive. Ask the patient if he thinks his physical defects have hindered his occupational advancement or social life.

When assessing for *conversion disorder*, find out if the patient was under severe emotional stress before the appearance of symptoms. Also ask if he recently met anyone with symptoms similar to his. Note the patient's attitude as you listen to his answers. Does he show a bland attitude toward the conversion symptom and any consequent disability? Does he seek extra attention?

When assessing for *hypochondriasis*, look for exaggerated concern, an unrealistic perception of symptoms, or a preoccupation with

Continued on page 58

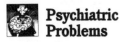

Anxiety-related Disorders

Other anxiety-related disorders—*continued*

serious illness. The patient likely will cite normal body functions as symptoms of a serious disease. Also take note if the patient conveys his medical history with unusually meticulous detail.

When assessing for *somatization disorder*, check for reports of illness extending throughout most of the patient's life. Vague or exaggerated complaints frequently recur over several years. In women, menstrual difficulty frequently constitutes one of the earliest symptoms. Note indications of anxiety, depression, drug dependence or abuse, frequent quests for treatment, or drastic changes in life-style in response to symptoms. Determine whether the patient has experienced interpersonal, marital, or occupational difficulties.

When assessing for *somatoform pain disorder*, ask the patient to describe his pain. Is it chronic and severe? Is it relieved by analgesics? Do any outside factors precipitate or worsen the pain?

Intervention. Because these patients usually won't agree to psychiatric treatment, your intervention may provide the primary therapeutic tool.

Give the patient support, focusing on his emotional well-being rather than any specific symptom. Listen to him, acknowledge his distress, encourage him to express his concerns, and focus attention on his personal strengths, assets, and accomplishments. Develop a trusting, long-term relationship. Schedule regular follow-up visits, rather than arranging appointments each time he experiences a symptom.

Try to discover how the patient benefits from his symptom. Have him keep a symptom diary. Explore together the connection between psychological stress and the onset of illness.

For patients in pain, consider decreasing reliance on narcotics by teaching alternative pain management techniques, such as self-hypnosis, biofeedback, and relaxation.

Besides psychotherapy, medical interventions include hypnosis and amobarbital sodium interviews. Although rarely effective in a general medical setting, confronting the patient with his problem may work in a psychiatric setting if done with care. Some patients receive successful treatment in multidisciplinary pain clinics with psychiatric practitioners.

Finally, be aware that patients with somatoform disorders may create enough frustration to make you want to avoid them. If so, acknowledge your angry feelings and seek help from a psychiatric liaison nurse or psychiatrist.

Factitious disorders

As the name indicates, these disorders are not genuine or spontaneous. The patient intentionally fabricates physical or psychological symptoms, starting and stopping them at will. While some patients enjoy complete control over their actions, others act compulsively. (See *Recognizing factitious disorder*.)

Frequently haunted by a painful past, the individual psychologically needs to assume the patient role. He may have had alcoholic, chron-

Anxiety-related Disorders

Recognizing factitious disorder

This chart will help you to distinguish factitious disorder from two somatoform disorders that produce similar symptoms—hypochondriasis and conversion disorder.

Disorder	Onset	Pattern	Associated features
Factitious disorder with physical symptoms	Early adulthood	Voluntary	• Severe personality disorder • No apparent goal
Hypochondriasis	Adolescence, early adulthood	Involuntary, based on unrealistic fear of illness	• Anxiety • Compulsive behavior • Depression
Conversion disorder	Adolescence, early adulthood	Involuntary	• Triggered by stress • Secondary benefits

ically ill, or sadistic parents who deprived him emotionally. Childhood experiences may have distorted his ego and self-image. Because of a long-term history of unhealthy coping, the prognosis is poor.

Factitious disorder with physical symptoms. Patients produce physical complaints in a variety of ways. Their symptoms may be:
• entirely false (the patient complains of acute abdominal pain when he has none)
• self-inflicted (the patient injects saliva into his skin to produce abscesses)
• an exaggeration or exacerbation of a preexisting physical condition (the patient accepts a penicillin injection even though he knows he's allergic to the drug).

Onset often follows hospitalization for true physical illness. In the chronic form of this disorder (sometimes referred to as Münchausen syndrome), the patient devotes his life to obtaining admission to hospitals. When confronted with evidence of his factitious symptoms, the patient denies the charges or quickly checks himself out against medical advice. But he'll often manage to get himself admitted to another hospital the same day.

The quest for hospitalization leads patients with factitious disorder to new cities, states, and even continents. Eventually, many are exposed. An acquaintance from an earlier hospital stay may recognize the patient, or one hospital may contact another for information and learn of past admissions for factitious symptoms.

Patients often abuse drugs, particularly analgesics and sedatives. They can't maintain steady employment, family ties, or lasting interpersonal relationships. Complications may include iatrogenically induced physical conditions, such as the formation of scar tissue from unnecessary surgery (gridiron abdomen), abscesses from numerous injections, and adverse drug reactions. Occasionally, a patient will spend time in jail for vagrancy or for assault during a psychiatric hospital stay, having been transferred upon the discovery of the true nature of his symptoms. (See *Features of factitious disorder,* page 60.)

Predisposing factors may include:
• serious physical disorders during childhood or adolescence that required extensive medical treatment and hospitalization

Continued on page 60

Anxiety-related Disorders

Features of factitious disorder

Patients with factitious disorder with physical symptoms exhibit a variety of unusual characteristics.

Pathologic lying
Uncontrollable, pathologic liars, patients will tell unbelievable stories. The patient may, for example, claim to be a undercover agent who was captured by the Russians or the illegitimate daughter of a famous rock star. Patients also relate their medical history with theatrical flair, but turn vague and inconsistent if pressed for details.

Repeated treatment
Patients actively seek health care and report being treated at many hospitals, sometimes hundreds or even thousands of miles apart. Evidence to support these claims might include gridiron abdomen, cranial burr holes, collapsed veins, and scars from self-inflicted wounds. But the patient's version of his medical history will be grossly distorted. You will not be able to verify many of his hospitalizations. Some patients will show souvenirs from past hospitals, such as identification bracelets.

Medical sophistication
Patients display remarkable familiarity with medical terms and jargon. The patient may ask for medications "on a p.r.n. basis" or insist on undergoing a barium swallow or a computed tomography scan. He may also give textbook descriptions of his symptoms.

Disruptive behavior
Patients disrupt hospital units, disobey rules, and demand staff attention. They frequently shift the focus of their complaints from one body system to another, requiring endless consultations with numerous specialists. For example, a patient admitted for chest pain might suddenly develop unexplained fevers or bleeding. The patient is usually willing to endure any number of invasive procedures, but may suddenly request discharge against medical advice. The doctor may order a psychiatric consultation once the patient's behavior becomes unmanageable.

Demands for medication
Patients frequently demand analgesics such as meperidine (Demerol), morphine (Duramorph PF), and codeine.

Infrequent visitors
Patients have few visitors despite prolonged hospitalizations. When visitors do come, they're often accomplices who restock whatever paraphernalia the patient requires to continue inflicting his symptoms.

Other anxiety-related disorders—*continued*

• hostility against the medical profession, sometimes caused by poor care
• underlying dependent, exploitative, or self-defeating personality traits
• a term of employment as a medical paraprofessional
• a significant emotional relationship with a doctor in the past or seduction by a doctor during childhood or adolescence.

Some researchers describe the disorder as common but rarely recognized. Others claim that it is rare and overreported because each patient visits many different doctors and hospitals, often using assumed names.

Factitious disorder with psychological symptoms. Patients with this disorder produce or feign a complex of psychological (often psychotic) symptoms. These symptoms become more severe when the patient knows he's being watched. The disorder may be chronic or limited to a few brief episodes. Most common in males, it's especially likely in patients with severe personality disorder. The symptoms usually fail to conform to any recognized diagnostic category; rather they represent the patient's idea of a mental disorder. Chronic patients undergo frequent hospitalizations.

Many patients take drugs, including psychoactive agents, analgesics, and hallucinogens, to achieve a desired psychological effect. Patients may also combine drugs, producing some extremely bizarre symptoms.

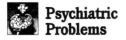

Anxiety-related Disorders

Drugs taken to simulate illness

Drug	Effect
Cathartics	Melanosis coli
Diuretics	Electrolyte imbalance, weakness
Thyroid hormone	Amenorrhea
Tranquilizers, barbiturates (in patients with allergies to these drugs)	Erythema nodosum
Self-injection of pentazocine lactate (Talwin)	Myositis, sterile abscesses, nonhealing wounds

Assessment. Limited only by their medical knowledge and imagination, patients with *factitious disorder with physical symptoms* may produce or feign a range of problems in any organ or body system. If you suspect factitious disorder, look for:
* multiple surgical scars at various body sites
* severe right lower quadrant pain associated with nausea and vomiting
* dizziness and fainting
* bleeding or severe hemoptysis
* generalized rashes or abscesses
* fevers of unknown origin
* lupus-like syndromes

When questioned, the patient may be evasive, hostile, or even threatening. Although he describes serious past medical problems, you may not feel entirely convinced. Expect the patient to display familiarity with medical jargon, look as if he is in pain, request analgesics, and demand immediate attention.

The patient will dramatically retell his medical history, but become vague and inconsistent if pressed for details. A complete history will probably reveal that he has deep-seated emotional problems starting in childhood. As a consequence, the patient lives with a crippled self-image.

When an extensive work-up reveals no medical problems, the patient will complain of new physical problems and manufacture more symptoms.

Many patients produce physical symptoms by taking medication. (See *Drugs taken to simulate illness*.) If a patient has hematuria, for example, ask the doctor to order blood studies to find out if the patient's taking anticoagulants. Repeated blood studies confirming the patient took such medication likely indicate a factitious disorder.

While the patient's undergoing a diagnostic procedure, you may request permission to have members of the health care team search in his room for evidence of drug misuse, contaminated bandages, or other signs of factitious disorder.

When assessing for *factitious disorder with psychological symptoms*, take note if the patient:
* complains of recent or remote memory loss, auditory or visual hallucinations, or dissociative or conversion disorder symptoms
* admits too readily to any other symptoms you mention
* responds to questions negatively and uncooperatively
* claims to be depressed or suicidal because of the death of a loved one. If possible, talk with family members or friends to confirm or deny this claim.

The patient may give approximate answers to questions. If you ask him to multiply eight times eight, for example, he might answer "sixty-five." However, a patient who is schizophrenic, exhausted, or simply trying to be funny will often give the same answer.

Intervention. Because the patient lacks insight into his feelings and has developed his symptoms to shut out painful emotions, expect

Continued on page 62

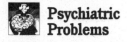

Psychiatric Problems

62 Dysfunctional Disorders

Anxiety-related Disorders

Other anxiety-related disorders—continued

many obstacles when trying to help. He might be especially resistant to therapy that attempts to bring out hidden feelings. When working with him, keep in mind the severity of factitious disorder. Although he'll be hostile and demanding, try to project warmth and kindness while remaining firm.

If you find proof that the patient's symptoms are self-inflicted, members of the health care team, including the doctor and the psychiatric liaison nurse, may confront the patient. If you're able to maintain a nonpunitive and supportive attitude, you may find that the patient feels happier and more relaxed once the confrontation takes place.

Help the patient become aware of the self-destructive nature of his illness. Try to make him realize that his illness represents a pathologic attempt to be loved, and to recognize his own cry for help.

Because the patient often may control his disorder, you may find yourself feeling angry and frustrated. If so, seek help from a psychiatric liaison nurse or psychiatrist in dealing with angry feelings. Consider exploring how your behavior may reveal your anger to the patient. Remember, anger will only keep you from understanding your patient's individual worth. If he knows you're angry, he'll withdraw or try to defend himself.

Keep in mind that, because the patient lacks effective coping mechanisms, anxiety and stress drive his behavior. Try to figure out what he gains from playing the role of patient, and try to identify the source of his anxiety. Help him focus on healthy coping mechanisms rather than on his complaints.

Self-test

1. Which most accurately describes anxiety?
a. an acute response to a definite, external threat **b.** a diffuse response to a vague threat **c.** an affective disturbance **d.** a sense of hopelessness

2. Drug therapy for generalized anxiety disorder includes all of the following except:
a. alprazolam **b.** phenelzine **c.** buspirone **d.** propranolol

3. The patient with a dissociative disorder may exhibit any of the following characteristics except:
a. losing touch with reality **b.** assuming a new identity **c.** aimless wandering to a new city **d.** reliving traumatic experiences

Answers (page number shows where answer appears in text)
1. **b** (page 26)   2. **b** (page 34)   3. **d** (page 46)

Mood Disorders: Depression, Suicide, and Bipolar Disorder

Margaret Benner, Assistant Professor in the College of Nursing, University of Delaware, wrote this chapter. She received her BSN and MSN from the University of Pennsylvania and her PhD from the University of Delaware.

Normally, each individual experiences a wide range of moods. But when an individual's mood becomes so intense and persistent that it interferes with social and psychological function (and the altered mood can't be attributed to another physical or mental problem), he probably suffers from a mood disorder. Mood, or affective, disorders represent one of the most common psychiatric problems.

The most current and widely used system for classifying mood disorders comes from the American Psychiatric Association's *Diagnostic and Statistical Manual of Mental Disorders,* 3rd edition, revised (DSM-III-R). DSM-III-R divides mood disorders into depressive and bipolar disorders. Suicide is regarded as a complication of depression. So, besides reviewing the two major mood disorders, this chapter covers suicide assessment and prevention. (See *Classifying mood disorders.*)

Depression

Affecting twice as many women as men, major depression is characterized by at least one 2-week episode of depressed mood (children or adolescents may exhibit an irritable mood). At some point in their lives, 15% to 30% of adults are diagnosed as having depression. Incidence is also high among patients hospitalized with medical illnesses.

Much controversy surrounds the cause of depression. Recent research indicates that it usually results from interdependent biochemical and psychodynamic factors.

Biochemical factors. Depression-related biochemical disturbances include impaired norepinephrine or serotonin transmission across the synaptic cleft. Sodium and potassium transport across cell membranes may be altered, resulting in sodium excess within nerve cells. What's more, levels of cortisol, human growth hormone, and thyroid-stimulating hormone may rise.

Sleep patterns. During depression, sleep and biorhythms are altered. In fact, studies of patients with depression have established four sleep abnormalities: loss of sleep continuity, reduced delta sleep time, increased rapid eye movement (REM) activity, and shortened REM latency.

Psychodynamic factors. Several psychodynamic models help to explain depression:

• *Psychoanalytic model.* Major depression results when hostile, ambivalent feelings, directed toward an early lost love object, turn inward. For instance, a child, unable to express his anger before others, internalizes angry feelings and experiences guilt. As an adult, his experience of a loss reactivates these feelings.

• *Personality organization model.* A child who experiences difficulty mastering developmental tasks develops low self-esteem. In later life, a severe blow to self-esteem will lead to depression.

Classifying mood disorders

Depressive disorders
Depressive episodes without manic or hypomanic episodes.

Major depression
One or more major depressive episodes.

Dysthymia
A depressed mood more days than not for at least 2 years. Depressive episodes are less severe and of shorter duration than in major depression.

Bipolar disorder
One or more manic episodes, usually accompanied by one or more major depressive episodes.

Bipolar disorder—manic
Dominated by manic episodes.

Bipolar disorder—depressed
Dominated by depressive episodes with at least one manic episode.

Bipolar disorder—mixed
Characterized by symptoms of both manic and depressive episodes and marked lability of affect.

Cyclothymia
Numerous hypomanic episodes alternating with numerous periods of depressed mood.

Continued on page 64

Mood Disorders

Drugs associated with mood disorders

Depressive episodes
alcohol
alpha-methyldopa
amphetamines
physostigmine
reserpine
sedative-hypnotics
steroidal contraceptives

Manic episodes
amphetamines
cocaine
levodopa
methylphenidate
MAO inhibitors
steroids
thyroid hormone
tricyclic antidepressants

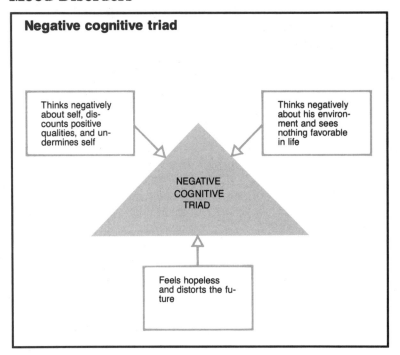

Negative cognitive triad

Thinks negatively about self, discounts positive qualities, and undermines self

Thinks negatively about his environment and sees nothing favorable in life

NEGATIVE COGNITIVE TRIAD

Feels hopeless and distorts the future

Depression—*continued*

• *Cognitive model.* In this model, depression stems from a negative view of self, the world, and the future. (See *Negative cognitive triad.*) An individual with this mindset views any loss, real or perceived, as total rejection.

• *Learned helplessness model.* An individual who's vulnerable to depression believes that he has no control over events and that no one will help him. Negative expectations lead to feelings of hopelessness and low self-esteem. He believes his behavior won't make a difference toward improving circumstances and blames himself rather than external factors for failure. As a result, the individual becomes passive and avoids change.

Precipitating stressors. In most patients, mood disorders, especially depression, represent a response to stress. Any major life event may cause depression if coping resources are inadequate. The greater the numbers and degree of stressors, the greater an individual's vulnerability.

Depression often occurs in response to a loss. The loss may be actual, anticipated, or symbolic. The depressed patient may have experienced:
• a change in body image and self-image because of medication use, disease, trauma, or aging (See *Drugs associated with mood disorders* and *Diseases associated with mood disorders.*)
• loss of dreams and fantasies
• failure to realize hopes and ambitions
• alienation or separation from a loved one because of death, divorce, or other factors (See *Dysfunctional grieving,* page 66.)
• loss of confidence
• reduced sense of autonomy and competence
• economic reversals, such as job loss, or social or interpersonal setbacks.

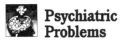
Mood Disorders

Diseases associated with mood disorders

Depressive episodes	Manic episodes
Collagen disorders Systemic lupus erythematosus	
Endocrine disorders Addison's disease Cushing's disease Myxedema	Hyperthyroidism
Infectious disorders Influenza Mononucleosis Tertiary syphilis Tuberculosis Viral hepatitis	Influenza Q fever St. Louis encephalitis Tertiary syphilis
Neoplastic disorders Abdominal cancers Cerebral tumors	
Neurologic disorders Dementia Multiple sclerosis Parkinson's disease Sleep apnea	Diencephalic and third ventricular tumors
Nutritional disorders Pellagra Pernicious anemia	

Note, however, that depression can be distinguished from acute reaction to loss. During depression, the patient experiences feelings of hopelessness, regression, self-criticism, self-deprecation, and suicidal motivation much more severely than during acute reaction to loss.

Assessment
You'll be able to recognize depression by the patient's evident dejection. Typically, he appears irritable, humorless, apathetic, lethargic, confused, and preoccupied with his own feelings. He often has little interest in his surroundings. Watch for slow, halting speech, with brief responses punctuated by long periods of silence. His limited conversation indicates a paucity of ideas. His difficulty in concentration indicates self-preoccupation. Most often he appears withdrawn and morose. Angry feelings directed inward and poor self-image cause the patient to neglect himself. Look for these physical characteristics:
• sad, dull expression, with a furrowed brow and a frowning mouth
• downcast, reddened, or tearful eyes, easily disposed to crying
• stooped posture and slow, clumsy movements
• unkempt, mismatched clothing, inappropriate for the climate or occasion
• dirty, disheveled hair
• general disregard for or disinterest in personal appearance
• poor muscle tone, dry skin, and an overall sickly appearance
• appearance of being older than chronological age would indicate.

Begin the interview with a broad statement and note how the patient responds. The patient's first words may indicate unhappiness or poor self-esteem. During the interview, he may express distress in

Continued on page 66

Mood Disorders

Dysfunctional grieving

Grief refers to a sequence of mood changes that occurs in response to an actual or perceived loss. Often described as a reaction to a loved one's death, grief may also represent a response to other types of loss, such as a change in family role, residence, or body image caused by injury. Usually, successful adaptation requires progress through the stages of grieving. Specific behaviors accompany each stage:
- *Disequilibrium.* During this stage, the patient undergoes feelings of shock and disbelief, followed by numbed sensation. He may cry and experience anger and guilt.
- *Disorganization.* Restlessness and an inability to organize and complete tasks characterize this stage. The patient suffers through loss of self-esteem; profound feelings of loneliness, fear, and helplessness; preoccupation with the image of the lost love object; feelings of unreality; and emotional distance from others.
- *Reorganization.* During this stage, the patient establishes new goals and interpersonal relationships. He begins to test new behaviors and expand his sense of identity.

Acute grief usually lasts from 3 to 12 weeks, with less extreme mourning continuing for 1 to 2 years. However, a patient who experiences *dysfunctional grieving* remains fixed in one stage for an extended period or has exaggerated signs of grief.

Besides, the patient who can't cope with change risks developing a *maladaptive* or *pathologic grief reaction.* During such a reaction, the patient may exhibit any of the following characteristics:

- excessive activity with no sense of loss
- physical symptoms similar to those of the deceased
- psychosomatic illnesses
- progressive social isolation
- extreme hostility
- wooden or formal conduct
- activity detrimental to social or economic well-being
- manic episodes
- depression.

Coping with grief

To help the patient cope with grieving in a positive way, take the following steps:
- Explain the normal stages of grieving, and tell him that the feelings and behaviors that accompany each stage are appropriate.
- Assess his present stage of grieving.
- Establish rapport and build trust.
- Convey an empathetic, caring attitude to encourage expression of feelings.
- Discuss the loss and concrete changes that have occurred.
- Encourage expression of anger. If the patient becomes angry at you, don't become defensive.
- If he's mourning a death or alienation from a loved one, encourage him to express his feelings and to review relationships that existed.
- Help him determine what realistic changes he needs to make.
- Encourage him to develop more adaptive ways of coping and make concrete plans for the future.

Depression—*continued*

a variety of ways. For instance, he may articulate his depression directly ("I'm feeling really unhappy"), descriptively ("I feel weighted down"), or with a metaphor ("A dark cloud seems to follow me").

When describing almost any situation, the patient conveys feelings of ambivalence and hopelessness. Nothing is any good. Ask about recent events and he'll select the saddest news to report. Other statements may express:
- readiness to accept blame for everything that happens
- disappointment with self, shame, and emptiness
- a sense of being a burden to everyone
- numerous apprehensions, especially fear of being alone
- excessive guilt
- feelings of uselessness, regardless of past achievements and contributions
- lack of faith in the future, for himself or for the world
- self-condemnation, no matter how insignificant his mistakes.

Note any indication that negative feelings occur with a pattern. The patient may feel worse in the morning with symptoms improving during the day or the reverse.

The patient may provide clues to his condition when he describes daily life. Unable to concentrate or make a decision, he frequently

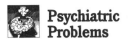
Mood Disorders

Signs of depression

Emotional signs
Anger
Anxiety
Depersonalization
Fear
Guilt
Helplessness
Hopelessness
Loneliness
Pessimism

Affective signs
Apathy
Approval-seeking
Crying
Emptiness
Irritability
Sadness

Somatic signs
Anorexia
Decreased libido
Diarrhea or constipation
Early morning awakening
Fatigue
Hallucinations
Insomnia
Muscle aches
Vague pains
Weight loss

Motor signs
Agitation or retardation
Seeking of physical contact or proximity

Cognitive signs
Focus on negative aspects of life
Loss of insight
Memory loss
Self-preoccupation
Slowed cognitive processes

Social and occupational signs
Apathy regarding work and learning
Decreased work capability
Social disinterest
Underestimation of competence

retreats from activities that, in the past, gave him pleasure. Depression has weakened his sense of responsibility and energy level. Important events are discussed indifferently. Take note if the patient mentions:
- losing interest in doing his job or caring for his home
- renouncing his religious beliefs
- breaking up once-meaningful relationships
- frequent fighting with friends and family
- an inability to feel or express love for spouse, relatives, or friends
- compulsive drinking or gambling.

Be alert for indications of withdrawal from social interaction. Often, low self-esteem contributes to a pattern of increasing isolation. Because he lacks confidence and fears rejection, the patient may be reluctant to interact with others. Also, he often focuses on his failures and guilt and tends to ruminate about past events.

Delusions or hallucinations may accompany major depression. Their content is clearly consistent with the patient's depressed state. For instance, the patient may anticipate punishment for a moral transgression or personal failure. Other delusions may focus on world destruction, cancer or other serious illness, or loss of wealth. Hallucinations commonly feature voices that reproach the patient for his shortcomings or sins.

Occasionally, the patient becomes agitated during the interview. He may pace about, making rapid jerking motions. He may wring his hands, cry without shedding tears, laugh inappropriately, or beg you to help him feel better. He may have picked at his skin so that it's scratched or bruised. At times, he may become mildly aggressive but probably will not harm others. However, the danger that the patient may act against himself is quite real.

Be alert for covert or masked symptoms. As emotional processes slow down, so do autonomic, neuromuscular, chemical, metabolic, and circulatory processes. The patient may develop various organic complaints. Because of the stigma attached to psychological disorders, many patients, especially elderly ones, deny their depression. In patients who are reluctant to admit to an emotional disturbance, such complaints as the following may provide the only clues to depression:
- anorexia or constipation
- dry mouth
- hypotension
- amenorrhea or decreased libido
- fatigue or malaise
- insomnia or early morning awakening
- headaches or vague aches and pains that rotate from one body site to another
- weight loss or gain. Usually, depression is associated with weight loss, but the anxiety that frequently accompanies depression may lead to overeating and subsequent weight gain.

Look for frequent infections. Depression also affects the immune system. The patient is more susceptible to colds, pneumonia, ulcers, urinary tract infections, viral infections, boils, decubitus ulcers, and other infectious illnesses.

Continued on page 68

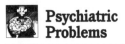
Mood Disorders

How signs of depression vary by age

Children
Physical signs usually provide the most important clues to depression in children. Young children often experience physiologic withdrawal. Older children often experience skin disorders, GI disturbances, headaches, and anorexia.

Children may be sad, irritable, readily disposed to crying, or vulnerable to phobias or frequent accidents. Depressed children probably experience low self-esteem and helplessness. Children may express anger toward parents or authority figures through acting out and rebelliousness. Such behavior may impair school performance and other activities of daily living.

Adolescents
When a stressful event precipitates depression, adolescents may experience signs similar to adults, such as flat affect, hopelessness, low self-regard, negative attitude, altered appetite, withdrawal, poor attention span, mood changes, and a loss of interest in usual activities. Adolescents may also show a marked change in physical or social activity or both, or an unpredictable behavior pattern. They may have outbursts in school or run away.

When depression has no apparent link to a stressor, predominant signs include anorexia, sleeplessness, disinterest in appearance, decreased productivity, feelings of worthlessness and failure, excessive use of alcohol or drugs, and possible suicide attempts.

Adults
Adults commonly exhibit the classic signs of depression. These signs may vary depending upon the severity of the illness.

Elders
In this age group, depression is associated with:
• feelings of uselessness and nonproductivity
• transition overload caused by too many life changes
• decreased human contact as loved ones die or move away
• physiologic reactions to medications.

The most common health problem among elderly people, depression often goes unrecognized because its signs are confused with the normal changes associated with aging. Common signs include apathy, sleep disturbances, fatigue, confusion, irritability, constipation, withdrawal, emptiness, nocturia accompanied by daytime urinary frequency, anorexia, epigastric distress, and somatic complaints. Elderly patients do not experience sadness to the same degree as younger depressed patients.

Depression—*continued*

Because anxiety often precedes depression, the patient may describe such symptoms as weakness, chest tightness, stomach cramps, shaking, dizziness, palpitations, lump in the throat, sweating, and diarrhea. Expect anxiety to increase as depression progresses.

The patient often fails to realize that his depression causes physical discomfort. Instead, he attributes feelings of hopelessness to the physical symptoms he must tolerate. The patient may express excessive and hypochondriacal concern about symptoms. Even so, because depressed patients are prone to physical illnesses, all complaints should be investigated.

Recent studies have demonstrated that depression impairs short-term memory and lowers performance on psychological tests. For this reason, doctors may mistakenly diagnose depressed patients as having a cognitive impairment, such as organic brain disease.

Biochemical studies. Numerous biochemical studies may help differentiate depression from other psychiatric, endocrine, or physical disorders. Although not yet widely used, you may encounter these tests.

In the *diurnal cortisol study,* serial blood samples are drawn from the patient at noon, 4 p.m., midnight, and 8 a.m. and evaluated for cortisol level. Variation in cortisol level among the samples may help differentiate between psychiatric and endocrine causes of depression and help guide treatment.

The *dexamethasone suppression test (DST)* involves giving the patient 1 mg of dexamethasone at bedtime, then measuring cortisol level

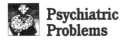
Mood Disorders

in six blood samples taken the next day at 8 a.m., noon, 4 p.m., 5 p.m., 10 p.m., and midnight. Blood cortisol levels between 4 and 5 µg/dl indicate that the drug hasn't successfully suppressed cortisol production. Uses of the DST include:
• providing supportive evidence of depression
• helping to establish the need for treatment of coexisting depression in patients with other psychological disorders, such as schizoaffective disorder
• providing relief to patients with excessive guilt who feel better knowing their depression has a physiologic basis.

Keep in mind that the DST has important limitations. For instance, a normal DST result doesn't rule out depression. In fact, if a patient with a negative DST result meets the DSM-III-R criteria for depression, the diagnosis will still be depression.

In the *thyrotropin-releasing hormone (TRH) infusion test*, the patient is given nothing by mouth (except water) after midnight and remains in bed throughout the test. At 8 a.m., I.V. saline solution is started, and the doctor injects 1 ml of TRH through a stopcock on the I.V. apparatus. After 30 minutes and again after 90 minutes, blood samples are obtained and evaluated for TRH level. Test results help differentiate depression from hypothalamic, pituitary, or thyroid disease.

The *stimulant challenge test* involves giving the patient 5 to 10 mg of methylphenidate twice a day for several days. If the patient reports any improvement of depressive symptoms, he might respond favorably to treatment with antidepressant drugs that have a norepinephrine-like effect, such as the tricyclic antidepressants.

Fasting tryptophan and tyrosine tests consist of measuring fasting blood levels of these two amino acids. Low levels point to either dietary deficiency or depression. Depression caused by deficiencies of these nutrients may respond to L-tryptophan and L-tyrosine.

In the *beta-endorphin test*, blood samples are drawn from the patient at 8 a.m. and midnight and evaluated for levels of this natural opiate-like hormone. Low levels occur in depression as well as in opiate and methadone addiction.

The *plasma serotonin transporter test* involves measuring blood levels of serotonin, which is associated with mood regulation. Low serotonin levels correlate with anger, aggressiveness, biochemical predisposition to depression, and suicidal ideation.

Noninvasive studies. *EEG sleep studies* involve measuring the onset and duration of REM sleep. Although not practical for most depressed patients, these studies provide clues to the pathophysiology of depression and patients' responses to antidepressant drugs.

Psychological tests. Various tests help assess the type and depth of emotions associated with depression. The two most commonly used tools are the *Beck Depression Inventory*, which evaluates the severity of symptoms commonly linked to depression (such as sadness, pessimism, and dissatisfaction), and *Zung's Self-rating Depression Inventory*, in which patients respond in writing to survey

Continued on page 70

Mood Disorders

Sample nursing care plan: Depression

Nursing diagnosis	Expected outcomes
Powerlessness; related to feelings of helplessness	The patient will: • state choices that will enable him to maintain control over life situations. • express feelings regarding problems over which he has no control. • explain problem-solving techniques that will enable him to function more effectively.
Nursing interventions • Develop a trusting nurse-patient relationship by being empathetic, caring, and honest and by keeping all promises. • Allow the patient to express his feelings openly by conveying an accepting attitude. • Help the patient to set realistic goals. • Encourage the patient to take responsibility for self-care practices and to develop a schedule for self-care activities. • Assist the patient to identify aspects of life he can control. • Conversely, help the patient identify aspects of life he can't control. Allow patient to express his feelings regarding this reality. • Encourage the patient to participate in activities that will help him develop a sense of achievement. Provide positive reinforcement for his participation.	**Discharge planning** • Review care plan with the patient. • Consult with a psychiatric liaison nurse or community health nurse to provide follow-up care, as needed. • Arrange an appointment with a psychotherapist to provide continuing care, if necessary.

Depression—*continued*

questions, solving the often difficult problem of eliciting verbal responses from depressed patients. Other tests include the *Hamilton Rating Scale*, which rates the severity of symptoms from information provided in the patient interview, the *Young Loneliness Scale*, which assesses absence of friendships and intimate ties, the *Dysfunctional Attitude Scale*, which assesses underlying maladaptive attitudes or assumptions, and the *Minnesota Multiphasic Personality Inventory*.

Planning

Before determining your nursing care plan, develop the nursing diagnosis by identifying the patient's actual or potential problem, then relating it to its cause. Possible nursing diagnoses for a patient with depression include:

• grieving, dysfunctional; related to loss of a cherished belief or value

• powerlessness; related to feelings of helplessness

• nutrition, altered (less than body requirements); related to loss of appetite

• self-esteem, disturbance in; related to numerous failures

• sleep pattern disturbance; related to depressed mood

• social isolation; related to depressed mood and feelings of worthlessness

• thought processes, altered (delusional thinking); related to low self-esteem

• violence, potential for (self-directed); related to hopelessness and unchannelled aggressive impulses.

Mood Disorders

The sample nursing care plan on the opposite page shows expected outcomes, nursing interventions, and discharge planning for one of the nursing diagnoses listed above. However, you'll want to individualize your care plan to meet the specific needs of your patient.

Intervention

Treatment includes drug therapy, electroconvulsive therapy, and individual, family, or group psychotherapy. The specific treatment selected depends on the severity of illness and the available resources. A combination of treatment methods usually produces the best results.

Drug therapy. For many patients, antidepressant drugs help relieve symptoms of depression. However, they don't correct the underlying cause, and thorough assessment of what caused the depression should precede their use. Patients may receive tricyclic antidepressants, monoamine oxidase inhibitors, or tetracyclic antidepressants. (See *Reviewing antidepressant drugs,* page 72.)

Tricyclic antidepressants (TCAs). Because of their effectiveness and relatively mild adverse effects, TCAs have become the drugs of choice for treating most types of depression, replacing amphetamines and other psychomotor stimulants. The most widely used TCAs include amitriptyline, amoxapine, desipramine, doxepin, imipramine, nortriptyline, protriptyline, and trimipramine. These drugs apparently relieve depressive symptoms by increasing the synaptic concentration of norepinephrine or serotonin, or both, by blocking their reuptake by the presynaptic neurons. TCAs produce sedative effects within a few hours after oral administration, and antidepressant effects within 7 to 10 days. This delay results from the drugs' slow effects on neurotransmitter metabolism. Be sure to explain to the patient that the drug's full therapeutic effect may not occur for several weeks.

Because of TCAs' delayed effects, a severely depressed patient may be at a greater risk for attempting suicide during initial drug therapy. Suicide risk also may rise as TCAs begin to take effect and energy level increases. For these reasons, a patient with suicidal tendencies generally receives TCAs in closely supervised psychiatric hospital settings only. Also, don't withdraw the drug abruptly. Instead, gradually reduce the dosage to avoid rebound effects and other adverse reactions.

To minimize such common adverse reactions as sedation and anticholinergic effects, you may administer TCAs in a single dose at bedtime. Such an administration schedule also may benefit patients experiencing sleep disturbances. To avoid serious drug interactions, such as severe excitation, hyperpyrexia, and convulsions, do not administer TCAs with monoamine oxidase inhibitors.

Monoamine oxidase (MAO) inhibitors. MAO inhibitors—isocarboxazid, phenelzine, and tranylcypromine—may help patients who don't respond to other forms of antidepressant therapy. Because these drugs may cause severe reactions, doctors usually won't order them until after trying two different TCAs.

Continued on page 72

Mood Disorders

Reviewing antidepressant drugs

Classification	Drug	Average adult daily dosage	Adverse reactions
Tricyclic antidepressants (TCAs)	amitriptyline hydrochloride	75 to 300 mg	Dry mouth, dysrhythmias, headache, mydriasis, tinnitis, seizures
	amoxapine	50 to 300 mg	Blurred vision, dry mouth, dysrhythmias, nervousness, peripheral neuropathy, seizures, weakness
	desipramine hydrochloride	50 to 300 mg	Dry mouth, dysrhythmias, EKG changes, extrapyramidal symptoms, increased ocular pressure, seizures
	doxepin hydrochloride	75 to 150 mg	Anorexia, constipation, dry mouth, dysrhythmias, excitation, palpitations
	imipramine hydrochloride	75 to 300 mg	Dry mouth, hypersensitivity, myocardial infarction, seizures, tremors, urinary retention
	nortriptyline hydrochloride	50 to 100 mg	Drowsiness, EKG changes, heart block, paralytic ileus, photosensitivity, sweating
	trimipramine maleate	75 to 200 mg	Congestive heart failure, dry mouth, extrapyramidal symptoms, hypersensitivity, mydriasis, tachycardia
Tetracyclic antidepressants	maprotiline hydrochloride	50 to 225 mg	Excitation, heart block, hypersensitivity, mydriasis, palpitations, seizures (high incidence)
Monoamine oxidase inhibitors (MAO inhibitors)	isocarboxazid	10 to 50 mg	Abdominal pain, discolored urine, dry mouth, dysrhythmias, hyperreflexia, muscle twitching, paradoxical hypertension
	phenelzine sulfate	15 to 75 mg	Fatigue, mania, memory impairment, nervousness, orthostatic hypotension, weight changes
	tranylcypromine	10 to 60 mg	Dizziness, dry mouth, dysrhythmias, jaundice, peripheral edema, vertigo
Other	trazodone hydrochloride	50 to 600 mg	Drowsiness, light-headedness, insomnia, dry mouth, diarrhea, hypotension

Depression—continued

MAO inhibitors apparently relieve depressive symptoms by blocking the activity of the enzyme monoamine oxidase, which is involved in the metabolism of catecholamine neurotransmitters, such as epinephrine, norepinephrine, dopamine, and serotonin. The reduced MAO activity results in increased central nervous system (CNS) concentration of these neurotransmitters.

Both isocarboxazid and phenelzine have a delayed therapeutic effect, with the patient showing improvement only after several weeks or months of therapy. Drug effects may continue for up to 3 weeks after discontinuation of therapy. In contrast, tranylcypromine usually produces therapeutic affects within several days, and MAO activity is restored 3 to 5 days after discontinuation. MAO inhibitors carry the same precautions as TCAs regarding administration to suicidal patients and abrupt discontinuation.

Severe reactions—some of them life-threatening—are associated with MAO inhibitor therapy. Paradoxical hypertension, for instance, can cause intracranial bleeding (possibly accompanied by a severe occipital headache that may radiate frontally), neck pain, nausea, vomiting, diaphoresis, dilated pupils, photophobia, chest pain, tachycardia, bradycardia, and dysrhythmias. If any of these effects occur, discontinue the drug.

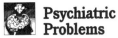
Mood Disorders

Hypertensive crisis may result from ingestion of certain foods and drugs during MAO inhibitor therapy. Amines (such as tyramine) or amino acids (such as tyrosine) may be decarboxylated in the body to form vasoactive substances (pressor amines) normally inactivated by MAO. (See *Dangerous interactions*.)

Tetracyclic antidepressants. These drugs—predominately maprotiline—are the most recently approved class of antidepressants. Like TCAs, they counteract depression by increasing CNS levels of norepinephrine or serotonin or both. Onset and duration of sedative and antidepressant effects are similar to TCAs.

Psychotherapy. Used alone, neither individual, group, or family psychotherapy has been proven particularly effective. Instead, psychotherapy is most effective when used with antidepressant drugs. It aims to help the patient (and, in family therapy, his family) gain better understanding of the illness and improve coping strategies.

Individual psychotherapy, a type of constructive interpersonal relationship, aims at alleviating symptoms and effecting a positive change in emotional well-being. Depending on the therapist's theoretical perspective, treatment approaches vary and encompass many forms of interpersonal relationships. All approaches, however, include the following steps:
• using verbal communication
• searching for a common goal
• mobilizing the patient's hopes and expectations of receiving help
• helping him to develop realistic expectations and to recognize that his problems aren't unique
• facilitating emotional arousal
• providing new information
• sharing in a set of principles
• fostering imitative behavior and helping him maintain improvements in behavior
• encouraging the patient in new social learning experiences
• developing an intense confiding relationship.

These factors help the patient to feel respected and understood and to develop trust in the therapist, so that he more readily reveals his innermost feelings.

Family therapy may be indicated if family members contribute to the patient's symptoms. In family therapy, the therapist attempts to examine how family members interact and to help the family reinforce the patient's adaptive behaviors and ignore maladaptive behaviors.

Group therapy helps the patient to modify his behavior by practicing new ways of interacting with others. Research supports the notion that group interaction promotes adaptive change. (See *How group therapy helps promote change,* page 74.)

In group therapy, each member's behavior within the group is examined. Because the group represents the larger world in which each member must function, helping members understand their behavior within the group may help them understand their interactions outside the group.

Continued on page 74

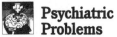

Mood Disorders

How group therapy helps promote change

All family and group therapy approaches incorporate basic principles. These principles help individual members—and the group as a whole—achieve greater productivity, competence, and an improved sense of well-being.

• *Altruism*—an emphasis on actions that demonstrate mutual caring among group members
• *Catharsis*—encouraging therapeutic expression of feelings—both positive and negative—within the group
• *Cohesion*—a shared belief that the group is meaningful to members and that members are meaningful to the group
• *Existentialism*—acceptance of the need for self-direction to help improve the quality of life
• *Family reenactment*—an emphasis on reliving early family experiences in a conscious, corrective manner
• *Guidance*—a group focus on making suggestions to help members modify destructive social attitudes and behavior
• *Identification*—adoption of functional behaviors and problem-solving techniques patterned after those of the group leader or other members
• *Insight*—an emphasis on understanding the causes of attitudes and behaviors
• *Interpersonal learning*—encouraging other members to describe or interpret events or experiences to individuals in the group
• *Instillation of hope*—fostering the belief that each group member can resolve his problems
• *Universality*—recognition that each individual's problems, fears, and emotions are shared by other group members

Depression—*continued*

Other groups that may include patients with mood disorders focus on such areas as growth, support, reality orientation, remotivation activity, and self-help.

• *Support groups* bring together patients and their families who share common concerns. By sharing feelings and experiences, group members offer support to each other while identifying better methods of coping.
• *Activity groups* aim to establish structure and provide direction for task accomplishment for regressed, withdrawn, or immobilized patients. Specified activities help patients cope with stress, develop awareness of reality, and enhance physical and learning abilities. Activities should enable the group members to experience a sense of accomplishment, sensory and cognitive stimulation, and interaction with others.
• *Medication groups* help patients understand why drugs have been prescribed, what they can expect from therapy, and what they must do to ensure safe, effective treatment. They promote compliance and help avoid rehospitalization.

Electroconvulsive therapy. Also known as electroshock therapy, electroconvulsive therapy (ECT) was first introduced in 1937 as a treatment for various psychiatric disorders. Today, ECT primarily benefits patients who can't take or don't respond to TCAs or other antidepressants and patients judged at high risk for suicide.

Contraindicated in patients with brain tumor, aneurysm, or recent myocardial infarction, ECT should be used cautiously in patients with peptic ulcers, cardiovascular disease, or glaucoma. In less than 1 in 10,000 patients, it can cause potentially fatal dysrhythmias. There is scant evidence to support the notion that ECT can cause brain damage, though a few individuals have reported prolonged or permanent memory loss.

In ECT, therapeutic effects result from inducing a tonic-clonic seizure by applying a low-voltage electrical current to the brain through electrodes placed on the temples. The patient usually receives a series of 6 to 10 treatments; however, this varies according to the severity of symptoms and the patient's response. Treatments usually are given three or four times a week on alternating days.

Although exactly how ECT reduces depressive symptoms remains unclear, it seems to produce biochemical changes in the brain causing increased levels of norepinephrine and serotonin. Before treatment, explain the procedure, including its expected benefits and potential adverse effects. Be sure the patient (or family, when appropriate) signs a consent form. Answer any questions and let the patient and family express their concerns. Commonly, patients fear being electrocuted or feeling the electric shock. By consulting with family members, you may gain their help in providing emotional support for the patient.

As ordered, prepare the patient for a complete blood count and urinalysis, electrocardiography, and in some cases, chest and lateral spine X-rays before the procedure.

Mood Disorders

To begin the procedure, the patient receives a short-acting anesthetic, such as sodium pentathol, and a muscle relaxant, such as succinylcholine. Administered I.V. in separate syringes, these drugs help reduce the severity of muscle contraction during the tonic-clonic seizure. The patient then receives 95% to 100% oxygen through a face mask. His chin is supported to ensure a patent airway. The electrodes are attached to the temporofrontal region and the electrical stimulus administered. This stimulus consists of 70 to 130 volts of alternating current applied for 0.1 to 0.5 second. In response, the patient experiences a seizure characterized by a tonic phase (facial twitching and curling of the toes) lasting about 10 seconds and a clonic phase (slight tremor) lasting 30 to 40 seconds. Muscular reactions may not be detectable.

After treatment, the patient usually sleeps about 15 to 30 minutes. Position him on his side, or turn his head to the side if he's in the supine position. Check blood pressure and other vital signs every 15 minutes for the first hour. Stay with him until he awakens completely; he may be disoriented and light-headed for up to an hour after treatment. During this period, reorient and reassure him as necessary.

The most common adverse reactions are temporary memory loss and confusion. Reassure the patient who fears permanent damage that these effects will pass. To decrease disorientation, structure the patient's time around routine activities. Assess for headache and nausea.

Nursing care measures. The following interventions may help accomplish the long-term care goals identified earlier.

Take steps to maintain adequate nutrition and ensure proper elimination. The patient may be unaware of physical needs or may have lost interest in eating. Because of inactivity, he's more susceptible to constipation. To prevent constipation and promote normal bowel function, encourage high-fiber foods and regular activity. Record daily fluid intake and output and calorie count.

A depressed patient may experience an increased desire to sleep, disturbed sleep patterns, difficulty falling asleep, frequent periods of awakening, or early morning awakening. For such a patient, keep a record of sleeping patterns. To promote more restful sleep at night, discourage daytime naps. Take steps to promote comfort and relaxation, limit caffeine intake, and administer sedatives, as ordered.

The patient's dismal attitude and self-defeating behavior often frustrate and anger staff, who respond by avoiding the patient, further increasing his isolation. If you find yourself becoming frustrated when attempting to help a patient, seek consultation with a psychiatric liaison nurse (PLN). The PLN's responsibilities include consulting with staff nurses who provide care for patients with behavioral, psychiatric, or emotional problems. She may be able to help you work more effectively with the patient and his family. She may also be able to help you deal with your own feelings of depression or burn out.

Continued on page 76

Mood Disorders

Depression—*continued*

Never underestimate the worth of your interactions with the patient. Remember that by establishing and maintaining a relationship, you're engaging in a form of individual psychotherapy. In many ways, you can help the patient begin to overcome depression.

Building self-esteem. The following interventions may help the patient develop an increased feeling of self-worth:
• Assist him with personal hygiene and other activities of daily living if he's unable to function independently.
• Focus the patient on small, easy-to-achieve goals directly related to his needs.
• Provide simple activities that he can easily and quickly accomplish.
• Offer praise for accomplishments.
• Minimize the significance of mistakes.
• Encourage the patient to take pleasure in personal strengths, assets, and accomplishments.
• Advise him to make a list of coping skills that enabled him to get through other difficult times. Identify how these coping skills might apply to his current situation.
• Involve him in decisions about his treatment. For example, ask when he would like his bath or what he would like to wear. A depressed patient is often indecisive; to help him, limit choices to two alternatives.
• Encourage him to make a scrapbook of pictures showing meaningful events, successes, hobbies, family, friends, or pets. Include in this scrapbook a list of strengths and accomplishments as well as inspirational articles and quotations.
• Encourage the patient to function more independently and assume control over life decisions.

Contending with negative thoughts. Help the patient to explore and express his anger, guilt, and other negative feelings. Listen carefully, without being judgmental. By talking with the patient, you may help identify the source of these feelings.

Teach the patient about his depression. Tell him that methods are available to help him relieve his sadness. Help him to recognize distorted perceptions and link them to his depression. Once the patient learns to recognize depressive thought patterns, he can begin consciously to substitute self-affirming thoughts.

When the patient's preoccupation with himself becomes overwhelming, promote diversion. Encourage him to indulge in pleasant sensations by taking a hot bath or listening to music. Try setting aside a specific, limited time for worry.

Grappling with guilt. Usually, the depressed patient's guilt feelings are disproportionate to past conduct. The patient expects too much of himself and needs to learn to accept human limitations. Don't discourage the patient from accepting responsibility for wrongdoings, but make it clear that excessive guilt isn't appropriate either. Discuss how seeking perfection and constant approval from others can create problems. Help him recognize the underlying conflict that may be causing guilt and assess self-accusations realistically.

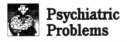
Mood Disorders

Offer these guidelines to help the patient learn thought-stopping techniques:
• Sitting in a comfortable chair, call to mind a single, unwanted thought.
• Once the thought forms, give the command "stop."
• Calmly and deliberately relax muscles and bring to mind pleasing thoughts.
• Practice this technique. Use it whenever self-defeating thoughts appear.

Be careful, however, not to criticize the patient for feeling guilty. Nor should you tell him to "just forget it." He can't do that. Saying so only makes matters worse.

Coping with loneliness. To prevent the patient from becoming isolated, try to spend some time with him each day. Avoid long periods of silence, which tend to increase anxiety. Discuss what you think the patient may be feeling based on your observations of his behavior. Because the patient may have slowed thought processes, speak slowly and allow ample time for him to respond. To convey a genuine acceptance of his feelings, avoid being falsely cheerful. However, don't hesitate to laugh with the patient and point out the value of humor. Discussing your own feelings of loneliness offers another way to convey empathy to the patient.

To help the patient cope with times when human companionship is unavailable, identify substitute activities that provide satisfaction, such as caring for pets, reading, watching television, listening to music, taking up hobbies, or regular exercise.

Use your relationship with the patient as a testing ground for human interaction. Point out both positive and difficult aspects of your relationship, and encourage the patient to express his feelings. Once he feels comfortable with you, encourage social activities. If the patient has poor communication techniques, you may need to help him learn new skills. Have him practice these new skills, perhaps by role-playing certain situations. Provide praise when he voluntarily interacts with others. Suggest ways the patient can increase human interaction, which include:
• initiating an activity with one person; for example, sharing a lunch, going shopping, or starting a simple conversation
• renewing a once-meaningful relationship
• doing volunteer work, such as coaching Little League or becoming a foster grandparent
• participating in groups, such as church or political organizations, exercise classes, or singles' groups
• reconsidering the opportunities at home for private, honest communication with loved ones.

Dealing with disorientation, irrational thoughts, or delusions. If the patient seems disoriented, spend time with him and reorient him to person, place, and time. If he's upset by irrational thoughts, teach him to use thought-stopping techniques. (See *How to control unpleasant thoughts.*) If he's experiencing delusions or hallucinations, the following interventions may prove helpful:
• Try to diminish the patient's anxiety and help him feel accepted. Constantly focus on reality, show empathy, and reassure him that you'll stay with him.
• Interrupt the patient's disturbed thought pattern. Decrease stimuli; convey that although you accept his belief the delusions or hallucinations are real, you do not agree with him. Discuss real events and real people.

Once you've established a trusting relationship, begin to help the patient recognize the delusion or hallucination and identify how it interferes with functioning. Encourage reality-based conversation, keeping statements short and simple.

Continued on page 78

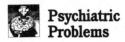 **Psychiatric Problems**

Mood Disorders

Depression—*continued*

Evaluation

Base your evaluation on the patient's expected outcomes listed in the nursing care plan found on page 70. To determine if the patient has improved, ask yourself questions like these:
• Is the patient able to make choices that will facilitate control over life situations?
• What feelings has the patient expressed over aspects of his life that he cannot control?
• Does he understand problem-solving techniques that will enable him to function more effectively?

The answers to these questions will help you evaluate your patient's status and the effectiveness of his care. Keep in mind that these questions stem from the sample care plan. Your questions may differ.

Suicide: Complication of depression

Depression may be the underlying cause in more than half of all suicide attempts. A depressed patient cannot engage in constructive problem-solving and often views suicide as the only way out of an emotional crisis. As depression worsens, he may become preoccupied with thoughts of death and self-harm. With any seriously depressed patient, your care plan must include provisions for preventing suicide and close observation for signs of suicidal potential.

Keep in mind that suicidal behavior encompasses five separate acts:
• suicidal ideations—thoughts about killing oneself
• suicide threats—either verbal or nonverbal indications of suicidal intent
• suicidal gestures—attempts to cause self-injury without actual intent to commit suicide
• suicide attempts—actions that could likely cause death
• completed suicide.

Evaluating variables. Studies have identified a number of social, demographic, and clinical variables that must be considered when evaluating suicide risk. (See *Suicide: Separating myths from facts*.)

Social variables. People from industrialized urban societies tend to be more socially isolated and more likely to commit suicide. Urban poor and homeless people commit proportionately more suicides than any other group. In contrast, family-oriented groups and cultures, warmer and more nurturing by nature, produce fewer suicides.

Demographic variables. Age, sex, marital status, and occupation affect suicide risk. More women than men attempt suicide, but more men succeed. One explanation: women tend to choose less dependably lethal methods than men. Adolescents, college students, and persons over age 45 are at higher risk than the general population. Higher numbers of suicides occur among single, divorced, and widowed persons than among married couples. Among married couples, the risk is greater for those without children. Unemployed persons have higher suicide rates than employed persons, though certain occupations carry an increased risk—most notably dentists, doctors, and police officers.

Mood Disorders

Suicide: Separating myths from facts

Many myths surround suicide. These myths may obscure important information that can help you identify and help at-risk patients.

Myths	Facts
A person who talks about committing suicide won't actually do it.	About 80% of persons who commit suicide express their intentions beforehand.
Suicide usually occurs without warning.	A person planning suicide usually gives many clues about his intentions.
A suicidal person fully intends to die.	Most suicidal people feel ambivalent toward death and arrange attempts hoping that someone will intervene to save them.
If a person attempts suicide once, he remains at constant risk for suicide throughout life.	Suicidal intentions last only for a limited period of time.
If a person shows improvement after a suicidal crisis, the risk has passed.	Most suicides occur within 3 months or so after the onset of improvement, when the person has the energy to act on his intentions.
Suicide occurs most often among the very rich and the very poor.	Suicide occurs in equal proportions among persons of all socioeconomic levels.
Families can pass on a predisposition to suicidal behavior.	Suicidal behavior is not an inherited trait, but an individual characteristic.
All suicidal persons are mentally ill, and only a psychotic person will commit suicide.	Studies of hundreds of suicide notes indicate that suicidal persons aren't necessarily mentally ill.

Clinical variables. Risk is greatest in patients who:
• have previously attempted suicide (lethality often increases with successive attempts)
• have physical illnesses that cause serious alterations in body image or life-style
• have chronic or terminal illnesses
• abuse drugs or alcohol (especially when actually intoxicated)
• are psychotic
• experience delusions or hallucinations.

Assessing for physical, emotional, and behavioral clues. Be especially alert when the patient:
• shows signs of anxiety, agitation, tension, loneliness, guilt, or helplessness.
• complains of nonspecific symptoms, such as fatigue, lethargy, malaise, headaches, and aches and pains. In one study, 75% of persons who successfully committed suicide had sought medical treatment for vague somatic complaints within 4 months before their deaths.
• undergoes a sudden mood change. For example, a patient who usually acts highly anxious and agitated suddenly becomes calm. Such a change may indicate that the patient has decided to solve his problems by taking his life.
• seems to be overcoming his depression. The patient now has renewed energy to plan and carry out a suicide attempt.

Continued on page 80

Mood Disorders

Bringing up a difficult topic

Patients may feel reluctant to discuss suicidal ideas or plans. So, ask about suicidal thoughts using any of the following suggestions to broach this difficult topic:
• "Sometimes pressures become so severe that people see no reason to continue living. Have you ever felt like that?"
• "If things got worse, what would you do?"
• "Have you ever felt so discouraged that you no longer wanted to live? Do you feel this way now?"
• "Have you ever felt miserable enough to consider suicide?" If the patient acknowledges this, say "Tell me about it."

To further evaluate suicide risk, ask:
• "How would you commit suicide?"
• "When would you do it?"
• "Do you intend to die or do you expect to be rescued?"

Depression—*continued*

A patient about to commit suicide may give several verbal and behavioral clues. Messages may be direct, such as clear-cut threats ("I'm going to kill myself. This time I'm really going to do it"), or indirect, such as giving away prized possessions or making veiled statements ("It would be better not to have been born"). Unfortunately, the clearest and most direct clue is an actual suicide attempt—which often succeeds.

Following through. Take any comments the patient makes about suicide seriously, and explore them further. If possible, ask the patient directly about his suicidal thoughts. (See *Bringing up a difficult topic.*)

If you believe a patient has a definite plan for suicide, try to elicit more information. Evaluate the lethality and availability of the method, the detail and concreteness of the plan, and recent preparations for death. The more potentially lethal the proposed method, the more likely the attempt will succeed. Risk increases further if the patient has access to the proposed method, and if the plan is well thought out and includes concrete details. A specific and potentially lethal plan calls for immediate intervention. (See *Assessing suicide risk* and *SAD PERSONS scale.*)

Acting immediately. Take steps immediately to prevent a suspected suicide:
• Make yourself available to listen. Respond directly to what the patient says. Don't reflect his questions back to him, as this will increase frustration.
• Provide a lifeline by calling family members or others who can help.
• Supply direct support. Do not give false reassurance that everything will work out. Let him know that while no easy answers exist, help is available and you will help him find alternative solutions. Get assistance from other professionals.
• Act definitively. Formulate a plan for follow-up and tell the patient what you want him to do and what actions you are going to take.
• Ask the patient to enter into a verbal agreement not to harm himself.

Inpatient psychiatric settings clearly spell out protocols and procedures for preventing suicide; general hospital settings, however, may not. In general, suicide precautions involve providing a safe environment by taking the following steps:
• Remove all potentially dangerous objects, such as razors, pantyhose, neckties, and glass.
• Initially have someone remain with the patient at all times.
• Accompany the patient to the bathroom.
• Keep the room dimly lit at night so that staff can easily observe the patient.
• Place the patient in a room close to the nurses' station.
• Lock all windows and utility and storage room doors; be sure windows are barred, grilled, or otherwise impenetrable.
• Administer all prescribed medications in liquid form whenever possible. If tablets or capsules must be given, check the patient's mouth to be sure he swallows the medication.

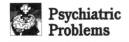
Mood Disorders

SAD PERSONS scale

One of the most popular and easy-to-use tools available to help assess suicide risk, the *SAD PERSONS scale* consists of the 10 major indicators of suicide potential. To use this scale, assign 1 point for each factor present:

Sex (males are more likely to successfully commit suicide)
Age (younger than 19 or older than 45)
Depression
Previous suicide attempt
Ethanol (alcohol) abuse
Rational thinking (impaired)
Social support lacking (including recent loss of loved one)
Organized plan
No spouse
Sickness (especially chronic, severe, or debilitating)

Total score ranges from 0 (lowest risk) to 10 (highest risk). This scale should be used as a guideline only; use your judgment and don't neglect unspecified factors, such as the patient's access to help and degree of hopefulness.

Assessing suicide risk

Use the following checklist to help assess the degree of suicide risk. For each item, an answer of 1 indicates a high risk factor, 2 indicates a moderate risk factor, and 3 a low risk factor. The greater the number of high risk factors, the greater the suicide risk. Use of this checklist should be tempered by your judgment and observations.

Alcohol or drug abuse
☐ 1. Continual
☐ 2. Frequent
☐ 3. Rare

Anxiety
☐ 1. High
☐ 2. Moderate
☐ 3. Mild

Attitude toward previous psychiatric help (if applicable)
☐ 1. Negative
☐ 2. Fairly satisfied
☐ 3. Positive

Coping strategies
☐ 1. Usually destructive
☐ 2. Occasionally destructive
☐ 3. Usually constructive

Functioning during daily activities
☐ 1. Poor
☐ 2. Occasionally poor
☐ 3. Generally good

Depression
☐ 1. Severe
☐ 2. Moderate
☐ 3. Mild

Disorientation or confusion
☐ 1. Severe
☐ 2. Moderate
☐ 3. None

Hostility
☐ 1. Marked
☐ 2. Moderate
☐ 3. Mild

Withdrawal
☐ 1. Marked
☐ 2. Moderate
☐ 3. None

Life-style
☐ 1. Very unstable
☐ 2. Slightly unstable
☐ 3. Stable

Previous suicide attempts (if any)
☐ 1. One or more of high lethality
☐ 2. One or more of moderate lethality
☐ 3. One of low lethality

Number of friends and family members available to help
☐ 1. One or none
☐ 2. Few or one
☐ 3. Several

Suicidal thoughts
☐ 1. Constant, with specific plan
☐ 2. Frequent, sometimes with specific plan
☐ 3. Occasional, with no concrete plan

• Closely supervise the patient during shift change, mealtimes, early morning hours, while he's shaving, and whenever a staff shortage exists.
• Do not agree to keep information about suicidal thoughts confidential.
• Ask the patient to contact staff for help if feeling highly anxious or overwhelmed.
• Assess suicide risk daily and adjust precautions accordingly.

Other care measures. Convey a caring attitude and place limits on excessive talk about suicide. Tell the patient that you'll discuss emotions but not previous attempts. Don't joke about death or belittle any previous suicide attempts.

Help the patient identify his positive qualities and provide an environment where he can better cope with his depression. Decrease environmental stimuli when necessary, and provide safe outlets for releasing emotions and anger. Review situations that cause stress for the patient and help him develop plans for dealing with them.

Encourage family members to talk with one another and develop improved coping strategies. Identify community resources and initiate referrals, as needed.

Continued on page 82

Mood Disorders

When suicide succeeds

A successful suicide attempt has more than one victim. Staff members who worked with the victim and other patients on the unit may experience anger, guilt, helplessness, and despair. Both patients and staff need to grieve and, if possible, to share their feelings. Other patients may become self-destructive, act out, or express anger at the staff for having failed the suicidal patient. Assure patients disturbed by the suicide that staff members remain available to help them.

For family members, societal attitudes regarding suicide complicate the mourning process. Friends, unsure of how to offer support, often do nothing. Self-recrimination and guilt may prevent family members from sharing their grief with others as they would if death resulted from natural causes. Family members may have mixed feelings, including resentment and rage, toward the deceased. If not acknowledged, such feelings can become chronic and deepen depression. Children often feel responsible for a parent's suicide and may experience depression, become preoccupied with suicide, act self-destructively, fail to grieve, or suffer from arrested personality development. Often, families avoid telling children the truth. Discourage this practice when possible, because it denies children the opportunity to deal fully with the death.

Bipolar disorder

This disorder is characterized by manic or hypomanic episodes. A *manic episode* refers to a period dominated by an elevated, expansive, or irritable mood that is severe enough to impair occupational or social function. Preventing the patient from harming himself and others may require hospitalization. Similar to a manic episode but less severe, a *hypomanic episode* doesn't cause marked impairment in social or occupational function or require hospitalization. Manic and hypomanic episodes don't occur in depressive disorders.

Patients with bipolar disorder will usually also experience major depressive episodes. In fact, they often experience two or more complete cycles of major depressive and manic episodes within a year. Patients may also experience mixed symptom episodes, exhibiting at once the characteristics of a depressed and manic state. (See *Seasonal affective disorder*.)

Patients with bipolar disorder are usually first hospitalized as a result of a manic episode. For this reason, we'll focus on assessment and interventions appropriate to the manic phase of bipolar disorder. But first we'll review some of the factors that may contribute to bipolar disorder.

Genetic factors. Increasing evidence supports the role of genetics in transmitting bipolar disorder. Several studies implicate a dominant X-linked factor. Bipolar disorder occurs twice as frequently in women as in men. Incidence among relatives of affected patients is higher than in the general population and highest among maternal relatives. The closer the relationship, the greater the susceptibility. A child with one affected parent has a 25% chance of developing bipolar disorder; a child with two affected parents, a 50% chance.

Precipitating stressors. Like depressive episodes, manic episodes in bipolar illness may be precipitated by a loss. One study found that more than 50% of patients with bipolar illness experienced (and were aware of) a significant life event before their first manic episode.

Biochemical factors. Just as lowered norepinephrine levels occur during an episode of depression, the opposite appears to be true during a manic episode. An excess of this biogenic amine may cause elation and euphoria. Other biochemical factors associated with mania include altered dopamine and serotonin function.

Psychological factors. According to psychoanalytic theory, bipolar disorder arises out of the patient's love-hate relationship with his mother. The mother receives great pleasure from the early dependence of the infant and feels threatened when the child matures and seeks increasing autonomy. She communicates to the child that behaviors that assert independence are bad. The child learns the necessity of meeting parental expectations, even at the expense of his own needs. The child resents the mother's demands, yet strongly desires to please her. This ambivalence disrupts ego development and leads to a punitive superego (depression) conflicting with a strong id (uncontrollable, impulsive behavior).

Mood Disorders

Seasonal affective disorder

Medical texts dating back to ancient times discuss the seasonal nature of mood disorders. Modern studies confirm this notion. Many researchers have shown a strong link between the seasons and the incidence of mania, depression, and suicide.

In addition, for many patients, mood disturbances occur according to a seasonal pattern year after year. The revised third edition of the *Diagnostic and Statistic Manual of Mental Disorders* (DSM-III-R) includes criteria for diagnosing a seasonal pattern in mood disorders. According to DSM-III-R, the patient consistently experiences onset of an episode of bipolar disorder or major depression during a particular 60-day period each year. Remission or a transition from depression to mania or hypomania also occurs during a specific season.

The term *seasonal affective disorder* (SAD) describes mood disorders with seasonal patterns. Research indicates that many SAD patients are women with bipolar II mood disorder (hypomanic and major depressive episodes). Onset of depression usually begins in October or November. The patient may experience somnolence, lethargy, carbohydrate craving, and weight gain as well as depression.

Researchers are also studying the relationship between the onset of depression in winter in SAD and shortened exposure to daylight. Changes in climate, light, and latitude may account for regular winter depression. Some scientists report that patients with SAD may benefit from manipulating environmental lighting, such as exposure to bright light during dawn and dusk. However, establishing the usefulness of light therapy requires further research.

Assessment

Psychologists describe the elation the patient experiences during a manic episode as the "denial of depression." This denial is a defense mechanism. The patient becomes elated to block out overwhelming feelings of anxiety, depression, and low self-esteem. As a consequence of this repression, the patient may become mistrustful and manipulative, fail to develop meaningful relationships, or cultivate independence to the point of seclusion. Other consequences may include damage to long-term success and feelings of omnipotence.

When encountering a patient experiencing a manic episode, you'll notice first his elevated energy level, increased enthusiasm, and euphoric outlook. The feelings of deep depression that underlie this surface elation may occasionally surface in bouts of sadness and withdrawal or outbursts of irritability and anger. Most of the time, however, the patient has little control over his incessant animation.

The patient speaks rapidly, laughs readily, tells jokes, gesticulates freely, and generally appears restless. Instead of focusing on his feelings, he may babble about work, love affairs, or social life. When you attempt to steer the conversation to serious matters, he may ignore you or become irritated. Watch for rambling and disjointed speech that switches topics with little or no logical pattern. Other symptoms may include grandiose thoughts, unrealistic generosity, seductiveness, and in acute cases, exhaustion.

Monitor your own reactions to the patient. Does he strike you as being superficial? You may like the person and find yourself enjoying his witty antics or energetic charm. But don't enter into a nonprofessional relationship. Remember the person needs your help.

The patient experiencing a manic episode often loves to write, and eagerly fills page after page. Don't discourage this—you'll receive important data for your assessment as well as help the patient express what really bothers him.

Other assessment clues may come from the patient's appearance. The patient may wear extremely bright clothing and jewelry. A woman may wear heavy, colorful, sloppily applied makeup.

Planning

Before determining your nursing care plan, develop the nursing diagnosis by identifying the patient's actual or potential problem, then relating it to its cause. Possible nursing diagnoses for a patient with bipolar disorder include:
- coping, ineffective individual; related to unmet expectations
- injury, potential for; related to extreme hyperactivity
- nutrition, altered (less than body requirements); related to excessive physical agitation
- sensory perception, altered; related to sleep deprivation
- sleep pattern, disturbed; related to agitation and excessive hyperactivity
- social interaction, impaired; related to hyperactivity
- thought processes, altered; related to biochemical changes
- violence, potential for (directed at others); related to anger.

Continued on page 84

Mood Disorders

Sample nursing care plan: Manic episode

Nursing diagnosis	Expected outcomes
Sleep pattern, disturbed; related to agitation and hyperactivity	The patient will: • sleep 6 to 8 hours each night without medication. • fall asleep within 30 minutes after going to bed. • deal openly with fears rather than deny them through hyperactive behavior.
Nursing interventions • Structure activity schedule to include established times for naps and rest. • Provide a quiet environment. • Assess patient's activity level and observe for signs of fatigue. • Dim lights and decrease stimuli before bedtime. To promote comfort and relaxation, administer warm baths, back rubs, or other measures. • Warn against consuming caffeine-containing food and beverages, such as chocolate, coffee, cola, and tea. • Develop a trusting nurse-patient relationship by being empathetic, caring, and honest, and by keeping all promises. • Allow the patient to express his feelings openly by conveying an accepting attitude.	**Discharge planning** • Review activity schedule and dietary restrictions with patient. Make sure he understands the need for adequate rest. • Consult with psychiatric liaison nurse or community health nurse to provide follow-up care as needed. • Arrange appointment with psychotherapist to provide continuing care, if necessary.

Bipolar disorder—*continued*

The sample nursing care plan above shows expected outcomes, nursing interventions, and discharge planning for one of the nursing diagnoses listed above. However, you'll want to individualize your care plan to meet the specific needs of your patient and his family.

Interventions

Patients with bipolar disorder may benefit from drug therapy and individual, family, or group psychotherapy.

Drug therapy. Lithium carbonate and lithium citrate treat bipolar disorders. (See *Reviewing antimanic drugs.*) Administered properly, these drugs can prevent up to 80% of manic and depressive episodes and reduce the severity of episodes that do occur.

Although lithium's exact mechanism of action remains unclear, the drug apparently alters certain neurotransmitters, affecting sodium exchange within the brain. Usually, lithium produces its full therapeutic effect within 10 days.

Because lithium has a narrow therapeutic margin of safety, preventing toxicity requires regular determination of serum levels as well as consistent dietary sodium and fluid intake. Initially, serum levels should be monitored weekly; once maintenance therapy begins, blood samples should be drawn monthly, 8 to 12 hours after the latest dose. Maintenance levels (usually 1 to 1.5 mEq/liter for acute symptoms and 0.6 to 1.2 mEq/liter after acute attacks subside) usually require a dosage of 300 to 600 mg P.O. three times a day. If serum lithium levels exceed 1.5 mEq/liter, the doctor will probably discontinue the drug for 24 hours and then resume it at a lower dose.

Mood Disorders

Reviewing antimanic drugs

Drug	Average daily dosage	Adverse reactions
Lithium carbonate Lithium citrate	600 to 1800 mg	**Blood:** Leukocytosis **CNS:** Tremors, drowsiness, headache, confusion, restlessness, dizziness, psychomotor retardation, stupor, lethargy, syncope, coma, seizures, EEG changes, impaired speech, ataxia, weakness, incoordination, hyperexcitability **CV:** EKG changes, dysrhythmias, hypotension, peripheral circulatory collapse, allergic vasculitis, peripheral edema **EENT:** Tinnitus, visual disturbances **GI:** Nausea, vomiting, anorexia, diarrhea, fecal incontinence, dry mouth, thirst, metallic taste **GU:** Polyuria, glycosuria, incontinence, renal toxicity **Metabolic:** Transient hyperglycemia, goiter, hypothyroidism, hyponatremia **Skin:** Pruritus, rash, diminished or lost sensation, dryness and thinning of hair

Lithium toxicity may develop when serum levels exceed 1.5 mEq/liter. Signs of toxicity typically include nausea, vomiting, abdominal cramps, diarrhea, thirst, and polyuria. Promptly discontinuing the drug usually resolves these toxic effects.

When caring for the patient receiving lithium therapy, warn the patient (and his family, if appropriate) to discontinue the drug and notify the doctor if signs of toxicity occur. Because restricting sodium intake increases lithium toxicity, instruct the patient to maintain a normal diet and normal salt and water intake. Because lithium may impair mental and physical function, caution against driving a car or operating heavy equipment while taking the drug. (See *Lithium therapy: Nursing intervention checklist,* page 86.)

Nursing care measures. During a manic episode, the patient needs to know that staff will help him control his behavior. Consistency and structure help provide reassurance; establish goals and clearly express your expectations. Sometimes, you may need to set limits on the patient's behavior. When doing so, clearly point out the specific unacceptable behavior, identify the range of acceptable behaviors, and suggest alternative activities.

The patient's behavior may disrupt and upset other patients. If so, plan activities that will help the patient express hostile and aggressive feelings without disrupting others. Exercise often provides a good way to relieve tension. Avoid competitive activities and activities that require a long attention span or fine motor skills. Attempting tasks that cannot be accomplished easily will only increase frustration.

Although the patient is usually not at high risk for suicide, his hyperactive behavior often increases the danger of injury to self or others. To help reduce this risk, remove potential hazards and all unnecessary sources of stimulation and distraction from the immediate area. If necessary, isolate the patient or administer prescribed medications as needed.

Limit organized activities to small groups. Moderate the number of activities in which the patient participates, depending on his level of tolerance.

Continued on page 86

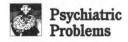
Mood Disorders

Bipolar disorder—*continued*

The patient in a manic state may need a high-protein, high-calorie diet and even supplemental feedings. Because he may be unwilling to sit down and eat, provide nutritious foods he can eat "on the run." Record daily fluid intake and output and calorie count.

The patient may require your assistance to promote rest and sleep. Help him by:
• providing time for rest periods during the day
• observing for signs of fatigue
• dimming lights and decreasing stimuli before bedtime
• using warm baths, back rubs, or other measures to promote comfort and relaxation
• prohibiting intake of foods and beverages containing caffeine
• administering sedatives, as ordered.

Evaluation

Base your evaluation on the patient's expected outcomes listed in the nursing care plan on page 84. To determine if the patient has improved, ask yourself questions like these:
• Does the patient usually sleep 6 to 8 hours a night without needing medication?
• Can he fall asleep within 30 minutes after going to bed?
• Does he deal openly with fears rather than deny them through hyperactive behavior?

The answers to these questions will help you evaluate your patient's status and the effectiveness of his care. Keep in mind that these questions stem from the sample care plan; your questions may differ.

Self-test

1. Organic complaints associated with depression include all of the following except:
a. anorexia, constipation, dry mouth   **b.** chest pain, dysmenorrhea, weight loss   **c.** fatigue, insomnia, malaise   **d.** headache, hypotension, vague pains

2. Carefully monitor a patient who is a suicide risk until he shows signs of overcoming his depression.
a. true   **b.** false

3. What characteristic distinguishes bipolar disorders from depressive disorders?
a. Depression is less severe in bipolar disorder   **b.** Patients with bipolar disorder wear loud clothes and change outfits frequently   **c.** Patients with depression respond better to individual psychotherapy   **d.** Patients with bipolar disorder experience at least one manic or hypomanic episode.

Answers (page number shows where answer appears in text)
1. **b** (page 67)   2. **b** (page 79)   3. **d** (page 82)

Schizophrenia: The Disordered Mind

Joan E. Mason, who wrote this chapter, earned her BS and MEd from Temple University in Philadelphia, Pa. She is currently a clinical editor with Springhouse Corporation, Springhouse, Pa.

Schizophrenia's chief characteristic is disordered thinking. Fragmented, confused, illogical, and bizarre thoughts shape the lives of affected patients. What's more, these patients may suffer from poor motivation, hallucinations, dull or inappropriate affect, altered self-image, and drastic changes in activity level. At some point in their illness, their work, social relations, and self-care will become impaired—sometimes to the extent that they'll require close supervision. (See *Frequency of schizophrenic symptoms.*)

Previously institutionalized schizophrenics are now being integrated into community settings, making it more likely that you'll come into contact with them. Helping them lead more meaningful lives requires patience and sensitivity; it also requires exhaustive assessment, development of a therapeutic relationship, and an understanding of schizophrenia's causes and symptoms. In this chapter, you'll find the tools you need to provide skilled care for them.

Theories of schizophrenia

According to European and Asian studies, schizophrenia occurs in 0.2% to almost 1% of the general population. United States studies, which use broader criteria and include urban populations, report an even higher rate. Researchers continue to debate the cause of this disorder, largely because of its heterogeneous nature. Most believe that genetics and environment influence its development, although disagreement continues about their relative contribution.

Genetic theory. Studies of families, adoptees, and twins indicate a genetic predisposition to schizophrenia.

Family studies. These studies indicate that the closer an individual's relationship with a schizophrenic patient, the greater his chances of developing the disorder. For example, children with one schizophrenic parent have a 5% to 6% risk. However, when two or more family members have schizophrenia, the risk of other family mem-

Continued on page 88

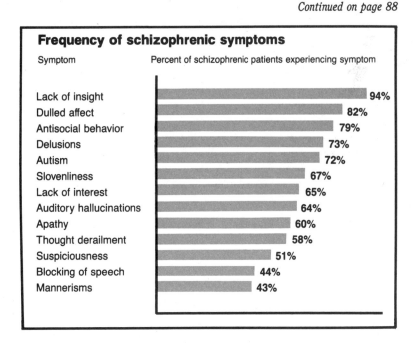

Frequency of schizophrenic symptoms

Symptom	Percent of schizophrenic patients experiencing symptom
Lack of insight	94%
Dulled affect	82%
Antisocial behavior	79%
Delusions	73%
Autism	72%
Slovenliness	67%
Lack of interest	65%
Auditory hallucinations	64%
Apathy	60%
Thought derailment	58%
Suspiciousness	51%
Blocking of speech	44%
Mannerisms	43%

Schizophrenia

Continued

bers developing the disorder rises dramatically: 17% for people with one sibling and one parent with schizophrenia and up to 46% for children with two schizophrenic parents.

Adoptee studies. Studies of adopted children provide stronger evidence of a genetic basis for schizophrenia: 16% of adopted children whose biological mothers were schizophrenic were at risk for the disorder. In the control group—adoptees whose biological mothers had no psychiatric disorder—researchers found no evidence of schizophrenia.

Twin studies. Because of greater genetic similarity, identical twins of schizophrenics are more likely to develop the disorder than fraternal twins. Over 45% of identical twins of schizophrenics develop the disorder compared to 14% of fraternal twins. However, because identical twins don't always share the disorder, genetic factors do not constitute the sole cause.

Developmental theory. According to this theory, schizophrenia develops if a person can't form strong interpersonal relationships. Freud believed that withdrawal of the libido (the sex drive) into the self leads to social withdrawal, narcissism and, eventually, hallucinations and delusions to compensate for lack of interpersonal relationships. Schizophrenic delusions provide defense mechanisms for the ego, and schizophrenic hallucinations represent wish fulfillment of unspeakable ideas rejected by the ego.

Interpersonal theory. Sullivan developed an interpersonal theory of schizophrenia, emphasizing the importance of the opinions of others in the patient's personality development. If the patient has few positive interpersonal relationships, he may develop a personality disorder or schizophrenia. Because this theory focuses on environmental factors instead of intrapsychic conflict, it's in close harmony with the environmental theory.

Environmental theory. According to this theory, both the family and physical factors may predispose an individual to schizophrenia.

Family influences. Although psychologists no longer believe that family conflict directly causes schizophrenia, the home environment may act as an important influence on the course of the illness or cause relapses in patients with chronic schizophrenia.

Earlier psychological theories emphasized the role of the patient's mother, blaming the disorder on mothers who were rejecting, cool, overly protective, or openly hostile. Other important environmental theories attribute the disorder to:
• a dominant, eccentric mother and a submissive, dependent father
• conflict and hostility between parents, which divides the child's loyalties
• parents who send ambivalent messages, causing confusion in their children.

Clearly, conflict frequently plagues families of schizophrenics. However, the relationship between conflict and the disorder remains ambiguous—family tension may result from the presence of a mentally ill family member or genetic factors.

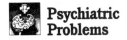
Schizophrenia

Physical factors. Studies suggest that a perinatal neurologic injury might lead to schizophrenia in someone genetically at risk. Schizophrenics often have ventricular enlargement, a possible result of perinatal injuries. Additionally, they have a higher rate of birth injury than the general population.

Viruses might also play a role in schizophrenia's development. About 80% of schizophrenics are born during the winter, when viral infections are most prevalent. High rates of diphtheria, pneumonia, and influenza coincide with high numbers of schizophrenic births.

Sociocultural theory. The notion that urbanization, social mobility, and poverty may cause schizophrenia became popular in the 1930s and 1940s. Because slum areas had a disproportionate number of mental hospital admissions, numerous studies linked low social class with mental illness. Researchers felt that poverty bred schizophrenia. In addition, the high rate of schizophrenia among immigrants indicates a sociocultural basis for the disorder.

In the 1970s, an alternative sociocultural theory—the drift hypothesis—became popular. Schizophrenics appear to drift down in social class as their disease progresses, gravitating to slum areas because of lack of motivation, poor hygiene, unemployment, and inability to function in a middle- or upper-class environment. This theory gained support because schizophrenics usually have a lower social standing than their parents.

Ultimately, however, schizophrenia cuts across social class and cultural lines, and researchers doubt that social disadvantages cause schizophrenia. More likely, societal factors accelerate or intensify schizophrenia in vulnerable individuals.

Neurobiological theory. Neurochemical or structural brain abnormalities may cause schizophrenia.

The most popular neurobiological explanation for schizophrenia, the dopamine hypothesis, suggests that dopamine levels at certain synapses significantly change in schizophrenia. Symptoms appear related to dopamine hyperactivity.

The actions of neuroleptic (antipsychotic) drugs provide the basis for the dopamine hypothesis. These drugs block dopamine receptors; the ones that produce the strongest blockade are also the most effective in relieving schizophrenic symptoms. Drugs that enhance dopamine transmission, such as amphetamines, exacerbate symptoms or may produce symptoms mimicking schizophrenia.

Receptor neurons contain at least two types of dopamine receptors: D1 (linked to adenylate cyclase) and D2. Most neuroleptic drugs produce much more D2 than D1 receptor blockade, which implies that D2 receptor hyperactivity may produce some schizophrenic symptoms.

Additional evidence for the dopamine hypothesis comes from postmortem studies. Researchers have discovered increased D2 receptors in the caudate nucleus and nucleus accumbens of schizophrenics, indicating hyperactivity of D2 receptors. Although this increase could result from treatment with neuroleptic drugs, increased D2

Continued on page 90

Schizophrenia

Continued

receptors have also been found in schizophrenics who hadn't recently taken neuroleptic drugs.

A new, precise technique, positron emission tomography (PET), allows direct measurement of the number of D2 receptors. In the future, PET will help assess whether schizophrenics who have never (or who haven't recently) taken medication still have excessive receptor activity.

The correlation between dopamine, neuroleptic drugs, and schizophrenic symptoms, however, doesn't prove that dopamine receptor hyperactivity alone causes schizophrenia. The biochemistry of schizophrenia may involve other neurotransmitters. For example, norepinephrine, serotonin, and gamma-aminobutyric acid may help alter schizophrenic symptoms, but studies of these neurotransmitters are sparse. In addition, the recent discovery of the importance of neuropeptides or cotransmitters has altered the concept of how neurotransmission occurs.

Regional brain abnormalities. Evidence suggests that some schizophrenics have structural brain abnormalities:
• Such techniques as computed tomography, magnetic resonance imaging, and PET indicate structural abnormalities, including those in the limbic system.
• Brain-imaging techniques and neuropathologic studies indicate some schizophrenics also have frontal lobe abnormalities.
• Many symptoms of frontal system disease resemble schizophrenia. For example, prefrontal cortex injury causes cognitive function disorders such as impaired attention, lack of spontaneity in speech, diminished voluntary motor behavior, decreased will and energy, and abnormalities in affect and emotion.
• One study of children of schizophrenic mothers indicated that the offspring who developed schizophrenia had larger-than-normal cerebral ventricles.
• Many symptoms of temporolimbic disease, including auditory hallucinations, disorganized speech, and verbal memory abnormalities, resemble schizophrenia.
• Dopamine affects a large part of the limbic system.

Although calling schizophrenia a frontal system or temporolimbic system disorder may be an oversimplification, regional brain abnormalities may indeed cause the disorder. After all, many cognitive functions are localized in the brain, so cognitive dysfunctions might be, too. Most likely, however, other influences act simultaneously.

Classifying schizophrenia
One important system for classifying schizophrenia divides the disorder into two types: positive (Type I) and negative (Type II).

Patients with *positive schizophrenia* exhibit better overall adjustment and functioning and normal mental awareness and ventricular size. Positive symptoms include hallucinations, delusions, bizarre or disorganized behavior, and thought disorders such as incoherence, illogic, derailment, or tangentiality. This type of schizophrenia responds well to neuroleptic drug therapy and is probably associated with increased dopamine receptors.

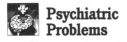

Schizophrenia

Five types of schizophrenia

The revised third edition of *Diagnostic and Statistical Manual of Mental Disorders* recognizes five types of schizophrenia, based upon signs and symptoms. The list below includes their distinguishing characteristics.

Catatonic
Drastic psychomotor activity changes from stupor to excitement, negativism (refusing to cooperate with simple requests for no reason), posturing, and stereotyped motions or mutism.

Disorganized
Blunted, silly, or inappropriate affect; incoherence; grimacing; unsystematized delusions; marked social withdrawal; hypochondriacal complaints; and other bizarre behaviors.

Paranoid
Anger, aloofness, argumentativeness, concerns about sexual identity or homosexuality, delusions of grandeur or persecution, frequent auditory hallucinations with a single theme, and retention of some functional skills.

Undifferentiated
Symptoms that don't fit other types or a prominent mixture of symptoms, such as delusions, hallucinations, incoherency, or disorganized behavior.

Residual
No prominent symptoms; signs of illness such as flat affect, social withdrawal, and bizarre thought and behavior patterns persist after at least one schizophrenic episode.

Patients with *negative schizophrenia* exhibit poor adjustment before the onset of the disorder, cognitive impairment, and structural brain abnormalities. Negative symptoms include obscure speech that conveys few ideas or information, blunted affect, inability to experience pleasure (anhedonia), lack of social contacts, apathy, short attention span, and poor response to drug therapy.

Studies suggest that schizophrenics with positive symptoms have an increase in vasoactive intestinal peptide in the amygdala, while those with negative symptoms have a decrease in cholecystokinin in the amygdala and hippocampus and a decrease in somatostatin in the hippocampus.

Researchers have devised a third class, *mixed schizophrenia,* for patients who exhibit symptoms of both positive and negative schizophrenia. The revised third edition of *Diagnostic and Statistical Manual of Mental Disorders* presents another scheme for classifying schizophrenia. (See *Five types of schizophrenia.*)

Schizophreniform disorders. First used in the 1930s, the term *schizophreniform* describes acute, reactive psychoses occurring in people with normal personalities. This disorder has active psychotic symptoms, isn't caused by an organic mental disorder, and lasts less than 6 months. Once the symptoms extend past 6 months, the diagnosis changes to schizophrenia, even if symptoms are residual.

Schizophrenia's course
Equally common in males and females, schizophrenia usually occurs in adolescence or early adulthood, but the disorder may begin in mid-life. Studies indicate somewhat earlier onset in males.

Schizophrenia may follow a subchronic course (lasting at least 6 months but less than 2 years) or a chronic course (lasting 2 years or more). Reemergence of psychotic symptoms (acute exacerbation) may occur throughout the course of illness. Many patients experience recurring episodes with incomplete recovery each time, producing progressive impairment. Patients may enter remission, but full recovery from chronic schizophrenia is rare. Certain symptoms, however, indicate a better prognosis. (See *Assessing the patient's prognosis,* page 92.) Because of an increased suicide rate and death from various causes, schizophrenics have a shorter life expectancy than the general population.

Assessment
Although schizophrenics exhibit many behavioral and physical problems, the disorder has no pathognomonic symptoms or predictable laboratory abnormalities. As with most psychiatric illnesses, diagnosis depends on patient and family history and meticulous assessment covering all areas of functioning. Behaviors and functional deficiencies can vary widely between patients and even in the same patient at different times. However, certain key signs and symptoms may alert you to the presence of the disorder. (See *Schizophrenia's phases,* page 92.)

Perception and judgment. Evaluate perception and judgment, especially during psychotic episodes. Schizophrenics characteristically regress to illogical and magical thinking patterns. They may

Continued on page 92

Schizophrenia

Schizophrenia's phases

Schizophrenia usually occurs in three phases: prodromal, active, and residual.

Prodromal phase

This phase is insidious, occurring about one year before the patient's first hospitalization. During this period, friends and family may report the patient has signs of a loss of will, inappropriate affect, and impaired job performance. Alcohol or drug abuse may complicate the patient's condition.

Active phase

Characterized by psychotic symptoms such as hallucinations and delusions, this phase marks full development of the disorder. The patient's symptoms are severe enough to alarm friends and family members and possibly require hospitalization. Carefully monitor the patient's physical and safety needs during this phase. Although schizophrenics who commit violent acts frequently draw public notice, research has yet to prove that these patients are more violent than the general population. Overall, the greatest danger is to the patient himself.

Residual phase

This phase resembles the prodromal phase, although dulling of affect and role impairment may be more severe. The patient may continue to experience psychotic symptoms but may be less troubled by them. In addition, the patient often experiences repeated, acute exacerbations of the active phase. Although the frequency and timing of these episodes is unpredictable, stress might act as a contributing factor. Impairment can range from none to severe enough to require hospitalization. Before a relapse into the active phase, the patient may exhibit such symptoms as restlessness or malaise (dysphoria), reclusion, sleep disturbances, anxiety, or ideas of reference.

Assessing the patient's prognosis

Characteristics	Good prognosis	Poor prognosis
Affect	Altered	Blunted
Age at onset	Older	Younger
Duration	Short	Long
Family history of schizophrenia	Negative	Positive
Marital status	Married	Never married
Neurologic function	Normal	Impaired
Onset	Acute	Insidious
Psychiatric history	Absent	Present
Psychosexual adjustment	Good	Poor
Social class	Upper	Lower
Structural brain abnormalities	Absent	Present
Violent tendencies	Absent	Present
Work history	Good	Poor

Continued

claim to be clairvoyant, telepathic, or blessed with a "sixth sense." Watch for indications of superstitiousness and ideas of reference (a distorted belief regarding the relationship between events and one's self). For example, the patient may believe television programs address him on a personal level or that he can stop traffic by blinking.

Hallucinations and delusions. Long considered the chief sign of schizophrenia, hallucinations refer to sensory perceptions that occur without external stimulation. The patient usually believes that the hallucinations originate in the outside world or in his body. Hallucinations may involve all five senses, singly or in combination.

Auditory hallucinations usually involve hearing noises, music, or voices. They constitute the most common hallucination in schizophrenia. The voices often comment on the patient's actions, argue with each other about the patient, or verbalize the patient's thoughts.

Visual hallucinations may include seeing flashing lights, objects, or people. Visions may appear smaller or larger than in real life, though color is usually normal. The patient may perceive a hallucination to be located outside his field of vision, for example, behind his head.

Gustatory and olfactory hallucinations may occur together as unpleasant tastes and odors. Tactile hallucinations include feelings of being touched or pricked, receiving electrical shocks, insects crawling under the skin, or manipulation or stimulation of body parts, especially sexual organs.

Note, however, that because these same hallucinations occur in at least 10% of other mentally ill patients, they're not definitive symptoms of schizophrenia.

Delusions refer to false beliefs that are inconsistent with an individual's culture, knowledge, and experience and that don't change in the face of facts. In schizophrenics and other mentally ill patients, delusions involve grandiose ideas, being controlled, somatic illnesses, or religious, persecutory, or nihilistic themes. The patient may sense the presence or power of someone not actually present. Take note if the patient relates any complicated plots, describes conspiracies, or elaborates loosely connected theories. Patients may

Schizophrenia

also try to involve you in highly abstract, usually twisted religious, philosophical, or political discussions. These discussions may leave you confused and exhausted.

Thought and language disturbances. Inability to discriminate among stimuli or to screen out unimportant stimuli may cause the patient to become overwhelmed and confused and to exhibit various thought and language disturbances, including:
• loss of the ability to form abstract ideas or make associations
• distraction
• concrete thinking
• misinterpretation of ideas
• looseness of association
• frequent digressions
• circumstantiality
• blocking
• perseveration
• echolalia
• obscure, metaphorical, or symbolic speech
• incoherent babble
• neologisms
• poverty of speech
• tangentiality
• stereotyped speech (speech that returns to same idea over and over).

Affect. Like depressed patients, schizophrenics show diminished affective responses. Patients become noticeably apathetic. Their facial expressions rarely change, and their movements and gestures lack spontaneity. They speak slowly, without expression, and avoid eye contact. Patients often describe themselves as emotionally empty and unable to feel pleasure, symptoms not unique to schizophrenia. In addition, they sometimes react inappropriately—such as by giggling when they learn of a relative's death. In an acute psychotic state, the patient may show intense, though often inappropriate, emotions such as sadness, rage, or fear.

Up to 60% of patients develop depression. Because of this overlap of symptoms, you may have difficulty recognizing depression. Some neuroleptic drugs also cause depression-like symptoms, such as akinesia (absence of movement), though symptoms often subside with dosage reduction or addition of an anticholinergic.

Motor disturbances. If left alone, schizophrenic patients may remain inactive for hours or occupy themselves with aimless, repetitive activity. In *catatonic stupor,* patients are fully conscious, but remain motionless, mute, and unresponsive.

Involuntary movement. Many schizophrenics exhibit some type of neurologic abnormality involving involuntary movements. Such abnormalities may include:
• stereotypy—repetitious, pointless movement, such as rocking
• mannerisms—normal, goal-directed activities, such as grimacing, that are odd in appearance or out of context
• echopraxia—imitating another person's movements
• automatic obedience—carrying out orders in a robot-like way.

Continued on page 94

Schizophrenia

Physical abnormalities in schizophrenia

Although schizophrenia has no physical symptoms, some patients do share characteristic physical abnormalities. Although some abnormalities may result from neuroleptic drug use, most were observed long before the development of these drugs.

Nonlocalizing neurologic signs

As many as 75% of schizophrenics exhibit nonlocalizing neurologic signs, including abnormalities in stereognosis (ability to identify the form and nature of objects by touching them), graphesthesia (ability to recognize figures written on the skin with a dull, pointed object), balance, and proprioception (ability to perceive movements and position of the body). These abnormalities probably result from defects in the integration of sensory information.

Ocular problems

Schizophrenic patients may avoid making eye contact or may stare for long periods. They may blink excessively and rapidly (60 to 80 blinks per minute when 6 to 12 is normal) or hardly blink at all. Scientists have consistently observed impaired smooth pursuit eye movement (SPEM), which causes problems with following smoothly moving targets. But because patients with other psychotic disorders exhibit impaired SPEM, its use as a biological marker for schizophrenia remains limited.

Vegetative symptoms

Schizophrenic patients may suffer from sleep, sexual, and body function disorders. Psychologists do not consider sleep disorders typical, though some patients show reduction in stage 4 sleep. Sexual problems occur more often—many schizophrenics have low sex drives and feel little pleasure during sex. Patients also experience chronic constipation, which can lead to megacolon.

Continued

Today, the common use of neuroleptic drugs may make it difficult to distinguish schizophrenic motor disturbances from drug-induced extrapyramidal adverse effects, such as tardive dyskinesia. (See *Physical abnormalities in schizophrenia.*)

Life-style. Assess daily activities. (See *Assessing self-care in schizophrenia.*) Patients may neglect themselves and become dirty and unkempt. They may wear ragged or inappropriate clothing and live in cluttered, filthy surroundings. They may behave in bizarre ways, hoarding food, talking to themselves in public, eating crudely, picking through garbage cans, and shouting obscenities on the street. Interestingly, research indicates that 50% to 80% of schizophrenics showed paranoid traits, eccentricities, or a lack of sympathy or feeling before their illness. But because schizophrenia begins insidiously, no one knows whether these personality problems predate schizophrenia or actually constitute early schizophrenic symptoms.

Social behavior. Assess the degree of social impairment. Schizophrenics often exhibit autistic withdrawal—they separate themselves from the external world and turn inward, preoccupied by their own fantasies. A disturbed sense of reality may frighten them into further isolation.

Approach-avoidance conflict. Usually introverted, schizophrenics shun the close personal relationships they inwardly desire. Their fear of rejection paralyzes them. Some schizophrenics use the image of watching a campfire on a cold winter night to describe their loneliness—wanting warmth, but fearing that approaching too close means getting burned.

To develop social skills and self-esteem, the patient must learn to associate with others. You'll need to assess his readiness for social interaction. Is he anxious and isolated in any social setting? Or can he tolerate a one-to-one interaction? Can he initiate conversations? Watch to see if the patient purposely avoids other people by staying in his room or by napping, reading, watching TV, or pacing. Does he respond briefly and then leave when other people try to talk to him? Some patients, especially those with paranoid symptoms, may try to discourage others from approaching them by acting aloof or superior, or by making threats or insults. When asking the patient about friends, try to assess the nature of his interpersonal relationships. Most schizophrenic patients have superficial friendships, if any.

Self-concept. A person forms his sense of self early in life, when he learns to distinguish between inner thoughts (self) and outer persons and objects (other). Some schizophrenics lose this ability to differentiate (loss of ego boundaries), which can cause severe regression. For example, a patient may fear loss of his identity by giving up personal possessions.

Although the patient might deny that he has schizophrenia, he's probably aware that he has a thought disorder, which also leads to lower self-esteem. He may try to delude himself and others with lofty statements.

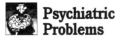
Schizophrenia

Assessing self-care in schizophrenia

Schizophrenia may interfere with such daily activities as maintaining proper hygiene and appearance, ensuring adequate rest, and urinary and fecal elimination. Consider the following points when assessing a schizophrenic patient:

Eating and drinking
□ Can the patient feed himself?
□ Does he act appropriately at meals?
□ Is his fluid intake sufficient to prevent dehydration?
□ Is caloric intake sufficient according to the patient's size and activity level?
□ Are suspicions or preoccupations preventing the patient from eating or drinking enough?
□ Does he eat too much, a possible indication that neuroleptic drugs have increased his appetite?
□ Has his weight changed?

Hygiene and appearance
□ Can the patient meet personal appearance and hygiene needs?
□ Does he dress appropriately?
□ Does he have fears or beliefs that prevent him from bathing regularly?
□ How much supervision does he require to ensure a proper appearance?

Oxygenation
□ Does the patient have any adverse effects from neuroleptic drugs, such as cardiac dysrhythmias, postural hypotension, or tachycardia?

Personal safety
□ Does bizarre behavior or a poor grasp of reality suggest that the patient might harm himself or others?
□ Does he hear voices that accuse or threaten him or tell him to do violent things?
□ Are neuroleptic drugs causing adverse effects?

Rest and activity
□ Does the patient get enough rest and physical activity?
□ Does hyperactivity or suspiciousness interfere with sleep patterns?
□ Do neuroleptic drugs affect motor activity?

Sensory and cognitive function
□ Does the patient have hallucinations, delusions, or other perceptual disturbances?
□ Can he interpret environmental stimuli and reality appropriately and respond to them?
□ Do certain stimuli upset him?

Sexuality
□ Does the patient have any bizarre ideas about his sexual identity?
□ Is the patient experiencing any adverse drug effects such as altered libido, gynecomastia, ejaculatory inhibition, menstrual irregularities, or lactation?
□ Does the patient perceive himself as sexually unattractive? Does he seem to have little interest in sex?

Urinary and fecal elimination
□ Is the patient experiencing urinary retention, a possible result of catatonic negativism or adverse drug effects (in patients with prostatic hypertrophy)?
□ Is the patient constipated, possibly indicating adverse effects of drugs on the autonomic nervous system, low-fiber diet, or low activity levels?
□ Is he incontinent or does he smear feces, both of which indicate severe regression?
□ Can he use the bathroom without being supervised?
□ Does he hide elimination products, an indication of depersonalization?

Goals. A schizophrenic often sets extremely high goals for himself, then never takes any steps toward achieving them. He may seem to purposely set himself up for failure. For example, he might say that he wants to become an engineer even though he has no plans to complete high school.

Environment. Evaluate the patient's immediate environment (for example, general hospital, psychiatric unit, or outpatient facility) and his family environment. (See *Assessing the patient in the hospital*

Continued on page 96

Schizophrenia

Interviewing the patient's family

To learn more about the patient's past, talk to his family as well. Questions to ask include:
• What was the patient's personality like before he became ill?
• What major life events has the patient experienced, and what were his reactions?
• What major stress factors does he face regularly?
• What led family members to finally seek psychiatric help for the patient?
• Did anything unusual happen at the patient's birth?
• Does the patient have any siblings? If so, describe their relationship. Where does he fall in the birth order?
• What was the last grade he completed in school? What kind of student was he? How did he feel about school?
• Describe the patient's strengths, interests, and activities. What are his career hopes?
• Does the patient have many friends? What are the friendships like?
• Does he date? Has he had any sexual relationships?
• What types of jobs has he held? How long did he hold them? How does he feel about work? What was his relationship like with employers and co-workers?
• Is there a family history of psychiatric illness, especially of schizophrenic disorders?
• Describe how family members feel about the patient's illness. What can you or other relatives do to help the patient?

Assessing the patient in the hospital environment

When evaluating the hospital environment and assessing the patient's well-being in the hospital, consider the following points:

Safety
☐ Is staffing adequate to allow one nurse per shift to provide consistent care and supervision for the patient?
☐ Are dangerous objects out of the patient's reach?
☐ Is a secluded, quiet area available if the patient needs to have stimuli reduced?

Meaningful activity
☐ Is the patient bored or inactive?
☐ Is the environment sufficiently stimulating?
☐ Are drawing, handicraft, and other materials available to help prevent the patient from withdrawing into fantasy?

Socialization
☐ Is the patient anxious in social situations?
☐ Can he tolerate a one-to-one relationship with selected individuals?

☐ Do you have enough time to develop a one-to-one relationship with him?
☐ Do you and your colleagues encourage him to interact with more people?
☐ Is a supportive group available to strengthen the patient's ability to interact and to provide learning opportunities?
☐ In a group setting, does the patient behave appropriately and interact with others?

Coping skills
☐ Does the patient have enough insight to recognize and cope with common life problems and return to the community?
☐ Does the community setting provide enough support in coping with anxiety, managing stress, developing social skills, training for a job, monitoring medication, and handling crises?

Continued

environment.) Questions to consider include:
• What stressors exist in both family and hospital settings?
• What opportunities exist for therapeutic and social interactions, growth, achievement, and the development of coping skills?
• Is the patient physically safe?
• Who does he consider to be his family and which family members does he consider important? This could be his nuclear or extended family, or the residents of a halfway house or a transient hotel.

During your interview, continually assess the patient's strengths and try to value him as a unique, worthwhile individual—this will help him learn to value himself. Look beyond the negative stereotypes associated with schizophrenia. The schizophrenic patient is often perceptive, sensitive, and a remarkably acute observer of human nature. Take notice if he's intelligent or humorous, or if he enjoys sports, music, or other leisure activities. Knowing the patient's strengths can help you establish communication. Express what you like about him and what you consider his strong points. (See *Interviewing the patient's family* and *Psychosocial assessment.*)

Diagnostic studies
Several studies, including brain imaging studies, tissue studies, functional and metabolic studies, and psychological tests, can help diagnose schizophrenia. Keep in mind, however, that diagnosis ultimately rests on clinical observation of the patient over time.

Brain imaging studies. Computed tomography (CT) scans may detect ventricular enlargement, which may be associated with poor premorbid functioning, negative symptoms, cognitive impairment, and poor treatment response in schizophrenics. They've also revealed sulcal enlargement and cerebellar atrophy. Structural abnormalities

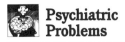
Schizophrenia

Psychosocial assessment

Psychosocial assessment should take into account the patient's background, family, social history, and sense of self.

Background
☐ What socioeconomic or cultural variables might affect access to quality care, compliance with care, or other aspects of treatment?
☐ Are community programs available for aftercare or vocational training?

Family
☐ Are family members optimistic and actively involved or pessimistic and inactive?
☐ What are the family's strengths and liabilities?
☐ Do family members expect schizophrenia to be easily cured by medication?
☐ Do family members believe that mental illness is a divine curse or a sign of evil blood? Do they have other misconceptions that might affect their ability to cope?
☐ Do family members anticipate being stigmatized or supported by friends, relatives, and community?

Social history
☐ Who does the patient identify as his main source of support, family or friends?
☐ What attitude does the patient's social group have toward his illness?
☐ How does the patient interact with others? Does he avoid people, maintain superficial relationships, or cultivate a few trusted friends?
☐ How well does he communicate?
☐ Describe his social history, including school, work, and interpersonal relationships.

Sense of self
☐ Can the patient distinguish between self and others?
☐ Can he evaluate the limits of influence of self and others?
☐ Does he view himself realistically or grandiosely?
☐ Is his self-image colored by gross distortion?
☐ How does the patient view himself in terms of goals and achievements?
☐ Does he use delusions of grandeur or other defenses to hide low self-esteem?
☐ What is his reaction to his illness and its effects (such as denial, resignation, acceptance, and feelings of being stigmatized).
☐ What are his strengths, and does he recognize them?

seen early in the illness suggest brain injury before the onset of symptoms, which explains why some patients don't respond to treatment.

Magnetic resonance imaging (MRI) may reveal decreased cerebrum size because of reduced frontal lobe size. It may also show cortical atrophy, widened sulci, and ventricular enlargement. (See *An image of schizophrenia.*)

Tissue studies. These have shown cellular changes such as gliosis in the midbrain, diencephalon, and forebrain—regions that contain major tracts of the limbic system, thalamus, and basal ganglia.

Functional and metabolic studies. Regional blood flow studies are used to investigate functional and metabolic abnormalities in schizophrenia. For some reason, blood flow to the frontal lobes doesn't increase in schizophrenics when they do tasks commonly thought to tap frontal lobe functions. Schizophrenics may also have depressed frontal lobe function, although this hasn't been proven. In addition, electrical brain mapping shows that schizophrenics have increased frontal system delta activity.

Psychological tests. Although extremely useful in providing information not generated during the patient interview or by the diagnostic workup, psychological tests alone will not confirm schizophrenia.

Psychometric tests can establish a patient's baseline intellectual functioning, making it easier to monitor progressive deterioration. The most common test, the *Wechsler Adult Intelligence Scale, revised (WAIS-R)*, measures verbal and nonverbal skills. A skilled examiner can piece together information about the patient's reasoning ability and ability to handle stress.

Continued on page 98

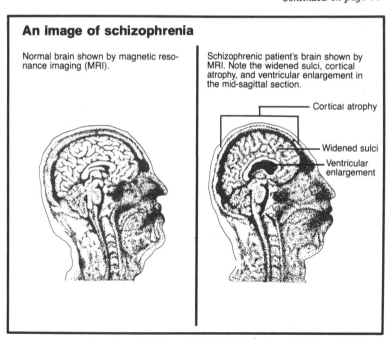

An image of schizophrenia

Normal brain shown by magnetic resonance imaging (MRI).

Schizophrenic patient's brain shown by MRI. Note the widened sulci, cortical atrophy, and ventricular enlargement in the mid-sagittal section.

Cortical atrophy

Widened sulci

Ventricular enlargement

Schizophrenia

Continued

The *Peabody Picture Vocabulary test*—one of several intelligence tests available for patients with special needs or for testing special functions—can help assess the verbal skills of non-English speaking, illiterate, or speech-impaired patients.

Neuropsychological tests assess cognitive, perceptual, and motor function as well as general mental ability. The *Wechsler Memory Scale*, the *Rey Auditory-Verbal Learning test*, the *Benton Visual Retention test*, and the *Wisconsin Card Sorting test* may help detect schizophrenia. These tests may show specific areas of impairment or a generalized deficit. Along with a history and neurologic examination, they may help rule out specific neurologic problems, such as brain tumor. If the patient has severely disorganized speech, assess for aphasic syndrome.

The *Minnesota Multiphasic Personality Inventory (MMPI)* analyzes personality traits characteristic of several psychological disorders. Unfortunately, the test's accuracy is questionable. Cultural factors may influence results.

Use of projective tests in diagnosis remains limited. Although schizophrenics show no set pattern of responses to the *Rorschach test*, some do have trouble focusing on specific parts of the test. Responses of paranoid patients may focus on persecutory themes. Patients with negative symptoms may show disorganization and poverty of thought.

Many schizophrenics tell stories of suspiciousness, persecution, or manipulation when taking the *thematic apperception test*—a projective test based on a series of pictures. Others show impoverished thinking or tell strange stories that have no relation to the picture.

Despite inaccuracies, the *draw-a-person test* remains popular. That's because some researchers believe that schizophrenics have a distinct style for drawing people. For example, people with paranoid tendencies often include knee and arm joints and large heads, emphasize the eyes, and position figures with a rigid stance.

Some researchers have used the WAIS-R with the Rorschach test to arrive at an index that allows objective and quantifiable evaluation of thought disorder. This index works best as a research tool, however. (See Chapter 1 for more information on psychological tests.)

Planning
When planning your care, focus on the patient's physical and safety needs, his psychosocial needs, previous levels of adjustment, and his response to medical and nursing interventions. Before writing your care plan, develop nursing diagnoses by identifying the patient's problem or potential problem, then relating it to its cause. Possible nursing diagnoses for a patient with schizophrenia include:
• anxiety; related to disorganized and delusional thinking
• communication, impaired (verbal); related to echolalia and neologisms
• self-care deficit (total); related to loss of touch with reality and apathy
• self-concept, disturbance in (self-esteem); related to apathy and loss of touch with reality

Schizophrenia

Sample nursing care plan: Schizophrenia

Nursing diagnosis	Expected outcomes
Sensory-perceptual alteration (hallucinations); related to excessive anxiety and loss of touch with reality	The patient will: • decrease his anxiety level. • report elimination of hallucinations.

Nursing interventions	Discharge planning
• Obtain consistent staff assignment, which allows for development of one-on-one relationship. • Provide consistent reassurance and assistance in interpreting reality (for example, "I don't hear the trees speaking Greek"). • Speak clearly, using simple, concrete terms. • Supervise simple reality-based activities, such as finger-painting or exercising to music. • Monitor effects of neuroleptic drugs.	• Consult with community health nurse or psychiatric nurse specialist to provide follow-up care as needed. • Review with family changes that have occurred while the patient was hospitalized and his future responsibilities at home. • Teach the family to identify symptoms that indicate a need to adjust medication or hospitalize the patient. • Refer the patient and family to a self-help group.

• sensory-perceptual alteration (hallucinations); related to excessive anxiety and loss of touch with reality
• social interaction, impaired; related to suspiciousness
• social isolation; related to apathy, autism, and communication deficit
• thought processes, alteration in; related to disordered thinking.

The sample nursing care plan above shows expected outcomes, interventions, and discharge planning for one nursing diagnosis. You'll need to individualize your care plan to meet the particular needs of your patient and his family.

Interventions
Ultimately, successful treatment for the schizophrenic patient requires a combination of medical, psychological, and social interventions. This includes paying careful attention to the patient's medication, developing a long-term relationship with the patient and his family, and seeking out community and vocational resources.

Neuroleptic drugs. Primary treatment for schizophrenia for more than 30 years, neuroleptic drugs appear to work by blocking post-synaptic dopamine receptors. These drugs reduce the patient's reaction to psychotic symptoms, such as hallucinations, and help to improve disturbed behavior. They also help to calm patients suffering from anxiety or agitation. In the United States, neuroleptics now include the phenothiazines, butyrophenones, thioxanthenes, indolones, and dibenzoxazepines; other drugs are available in Canada and Europe, and researchers are investigating still others.

Neuroleptic drugs differ in chemical structure, absorption rate, potency, distribution, and adverse effects. But because all of these drugs are remarkably similar in pharmacologic action and effectiveness, doctors usually prescribe only one drug at a time. In addition, all seem equally effective for all types of schizophrenia. So the choice of drug depends on the patient's tolerance of adverse effects, previous response to treatment, and his family history of drug response, instead of the type or severity of schizophrenia.

The first goal when treating acutely psychotic, highly agitated schizophrenic patients is rapid symptom control. Chlorpromazine

Continued on page 100

Schizophrenia

Neuroleptic malignant syndrome

Potentially life threatening, neuroleptic malignant syndrome (NMS) may occur with long-term neuroleptic drug therapy. Once considered rare, NMS strikes 0.5% to 1% of all patients receiving neuroleptic drugs, causing death in 20% to 30% of those affected.

Neuroleptic drugs block dopamine, a neurotransmitter, at specific receptor sites in the brain. Usually, patients compensate by producing more dopamine. However, patients with fluid and electrolyte imbalances, nutritional deficiencies, and organic brain disorders may be unable to overcome the effects of the dopamine blockade and thereby face an increased risk of developing NMS.

Hyperpyrexia constitutes the hallmark sign of NMS. Body temperature may go as high as 108° F. (42.2° C.). Signs of autonomic dysfunction include hypertension, tachycardia, tachypnea, diaphoresis, and incontinence. Severe extrapyramidal symptoms, such as lead-pipe rigidity, opisthotonos, trismus, dysphagia, dyskinetic movement, and flexor-extensor posturing, may also occur. Mental status changes may include delirium, mutism, stupor, or coma.

Treatment
Discontinuation of neuroleptics usually leads to recovery in 5 to 7 days. Drug therapy may include *amantadine* (Symmetrel), an antiviral and antiparkinson agent that alleviates extrapyramidal signs and hyperpyrexia, and *bromocriptine* (Parlodel), a dopamine agonist that counteracts dopamine blockade. *Dantrolene sodium* (Dantrium), a skeletal muscle relaxant, may be given to decrease muscle contractions.

Continued

(Thorazine)—100 to 300 mg daily—has long been the drug of choice, though use of haloperidol (Haldol) is increasing. For patients who don't respond to conventional treatment or dosages, doctors have tried several hundred milligrams of haloperidol or several grams of chlorpromazine, as well as electroconvulsive therapy. Although these treatments may be used as a last resort, they haven't been studied adequately and may even exacerbate central nervous system effects.

Drug therapy achieves the best effect early in the illness when positive symptoms predominate. Indicators of a poor drug response include chronicity and negative symptoms. Because many schizophrenics develop more negative symptoms over time, some function better without drugs.

Maintenance therapy. Patients who respond to short-term neuroleptic therapy make good candidates for long-term preventive therapy. Although maintenance doses of neuroleptic drugs can control symptoms in chronically psychotic patients, they also can cause irreversible neurologic damage. (See *Neuroleptic malignant syndrome.*) As a result, individually titrate drug doses and carefully monitor patients to be sure they're still benefiting from treatment. Patients who respond well to a drug in the acute stages of schizophrenia usually receive maintenance therapy for 1 year after the initial psychotic episode; patients who've had two such episodes may receive preventive treatment lasting up to 5 years. (See *Alternative drug therapy.*)

Electroconvulsive therapy (ECT). Primarily used for patients who don't respond to neuroleptic drugs alone, ECT provides rapid effects in catatonic patients and in patients with secondary depression. It may provide important, though short-lived, benefits in patients with acute schizophrenia. However, studies of ECT's effectiveness remain inconclusive.

Psychosocial care. The success of neuroleptic drugs in treating schizophrenia and preventing relapses may overshadow the value of psychotherapy, but successful treatment often requires both types of interventions. For example, the patient may suffer psychotic symptoms less frequently after receiving drugs, but may still require therapy to learn vocational skills or how to get along with others.

Traditionally, psychosocial care meant individual, family, or group psychotherapy. Today, it also means working with hospital social workers to help find community and government programs that provide food, shelter, vocational training, and health care. Unfortunately, many communities provide limited services at best.

Each patient needs individualized psychosocial care, depending on his living situation and phase of illness. For instance, one patient may need continued care in a hospital. Another patient, living at home with his family, might require family therapy, whereas a patient living alone might benefit most from the social interaction provided by a day hospital program or a visiting nurse. Usually, a patient's needs change as he moves from a hospital to a long-term group residence.

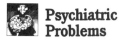

Schizophrenia

Alternative drug therapy

Anxiolytics and many other drugs help treat schizophrenia, but their usefulness isn't completely understood. Besides relieving anxiety, *anxiolytics* (especially benzodiazepines) relieve the motor restlessness associated with neuroleptics. High dosages have been used experimentally as primary antipsychotic agents, mainly to relieve positive symptoms such as thought disorder, delusions, and hallucinations. Although research remains inconclusive, anxiolytics may ease gamma-aminobutyric acid neurotransmission, which in turn may alter dopamine activity.

Commonly used to treat manic disorders, *lithium carbonate* (Eskalith) may decrease impulsive and aggressive behaviors, hyperactivity, excitation, and mood instability in schizophrenia. However, researchers have yet to make conclusions about the drug's effectiveness.

Antidepressants have been used to combat depression. Unfortunately, they are usually ineffective and may even exacerbate thought disorder.

Beta blockers, such as propranolol (Inderal), may be effective in high dosages (up to 3,000 mg daily). Propranolol raises serum levels of neuroleptic drugs, but this may not be its main advantage. It's also reported to decrease aggressiveness and outbursts of temper and, in small dosages, to lessen akathisia.

Carbamazepine (Tegretol), mainly used as an analgesic and an anticonvulsant, may curb aggressive behavior. *Clonidine* (Catapres), an antihypertensive, diminishes norepinephrine release by stimulating presynaptic alpha-2 receptors. Studies of its effectiveness yield contradictory results.

Individual psychotherapy. Despite its popularity several years ago, individual psychotherapy has come under scrutiny as treatment for chronic schizophrenia. Even so, a long-term, supportive, reality-oriented relationship with a psychiatrist or other professional can still help the patient develop new ways to cope, and identify stressors and prodromal symptoms of relapse. Occasionally, a patient may be able to explore his feelings about developing close relationships with others.

Group therapy. The notion that patients benefit from interacting with one another and their therapist provides the basis for group therapy. While group interaction can provide insight, it may actually harm psychotic patients, who frequently misinterpret stressful situations. Schizophrenic patients benefit most from a highly structured group with goals limited according to the capabilities of the members. Goals might include providing a supportive environment where patients can develop social skills and make friends. Patients who do well in group therapy when hospitalized often do well when treated as outpatients.

Family therapy. Living with the family may be a workable, albeit difficult, alternative for many schizophrenics. Be aware of the dangers brought on by rekindling old hostilities and dependencies. When the family becomes too emotionally involved, it can increase the patient's daily stress. Such a situation often calls for family therapy, which may help prevent a relapse, especially when combined with drug therapy.

Family members may also benefit from information on schizophrenia, including the importance of long-term care and what outcomes to expect. Education may help them learn to comply with the patient's treatment regimen and to avoid becoming overly critical or too emotionally involved.

Vocational training. Patients who lack job skills may benefit from vocational training. Simple repetitive jobs that allow some social distance, such as those found in sheltered workshops, succeed best at first. Eventually, patients may move on to more demanding jobs.

Some patients cannot maintain employment in any setting because of apathy, lack of motivation, or chronic psychosis. When possible, though, encourage patients to work. A job provides an opportunity to gain income, develop independence, improve self-esteem, and interact with others. (See *Milieu therapy,* page 102.)

Nursing care measures. By creating a trusting therapeutic relationship with the patient, you can promote long-range treatment goals and help prevent relapses. To accomplish this, coordinate your efforts with other health care team members.

Developing trust. Because patients usually expect rejection, building relationships with them is extremely difficult. Be prepared to have your sincerity tested often. Don't become discouraged by slow progress. You'll have to put aside your own need for personal acceptance. (See *Developing self-awareness,* page 103.)

Keep promises. If, for example, you have to miss an appointment, notify the patient ahead of time and explain your situation. To gain

Continued on page 102

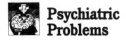
Schizophrenia

Continued

Based on the idea that a structured hospital environment provides therapeutic benefits, milieu therapy takes into account everything from the architectural design of the unit to the types of residents. Therapeutic elements include:
• a small unit with a high staff-patient ratio
• low staff turnover
• a small number of psychotic patients
• short-term admissions
• low levels of anger and aggression in patients
• a supportive staff with broad delegation of responsibility and clear lines of authority
• a problem-solving approach.

Patients may also benefit from the structure and discipline achieved through regular daily activities and rewarding appropriate behavior. Simple and consistent treatment works best. Staff should provide reasonable controls on behavior and allow patients sufficient personal space. Although patients may improve while in the hospital setting, they may regress after discharge.

the trust of a withdrawn patient who won't respond to spoken overtures, offer to share an apple or candy. Use touch, but be cautious; a suspicious patient might interpret touch as sexually aggressive or threatening.

Don't push a withdrawn patient to speak or ask probing questions. Instead, sit with him silently or talk about a neutral topic. In your talks, try to instill a feeling of hope. If the patient seems uncomfortable in a structured social setting, try to engage him in conversation while he participates in routine activities, such as taking a walk. Simple, direct statements, such as "I understand you're frightened, but I promise not to hurt you," help to reassure the fearful and regressed patient.

If the patient's distorted perception or bizarre behavior endangers his health or safety, approach the situation carefully. Tell him you're concerned, then take steps to ensure his well-being. For example, if the patient refuses to eat or drink, you might allow him to select his food, taste the meal first, or provide tamper-proof foods such as unshelled hard-boiled eggs or unopened canned goods or liquids.

If the patient requires restraint, explain that it is for his own protection. Also explain invasive procedures, such as tube feedings or injections. These interventions can interfere with building a relationship, so ask a co-worker to perform them, when possible.

Building communication. When building a one-on-one relationship with the patient, try to communicate feelings of nurturance and warmth and a sense of hope. Nonverbal communication such as sharing a snack may be a powerful way to demonstrate caring to the patient.

Upon hearing an incoherent statement, such as "The leaves are calling to me, go tell the prime minister," try to decode the patient's message. Let the patient know you don't understand him and encourage him to express himself more clearly. This requires patience, but ignoring the patient or pretending to understand him will hamper your relationship. Through persistence, you can often identify themes in even the most garbled speech, and this knowledge will help you reach the patient.

Controlling anxiety. Speak clearly and concisely, stay with the patient, and initiate activities that improve short-term coping and relieve tension. If the patient's anxiety or disorganization appears to be caused by his environment, change his surroundings. Learn to recognize signs of acute disorganization and increasing anxiety before a crisis occurs.

Reinforcing reality. If the patient experiences hallucinations or delusions, focus on the "here and now." Don't enter into a long philosophical discussion. Make it clear you don't agree with delusional beliefs, although you understand that hallucinations are real for the patient. For example, you might say to the patient, "You may think the trees are speaking Greek, but it's not possible." Express empathy for the emotional impact of the patient's false beliefs. For example, you might say, "I can understand your feeling scared and sad when the voices command you to kill yourself." Try to identify

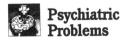

Schizophrenia

Developing self-awareness

Few medical diagnoses provoke as strong an emotional reaction as does "schizophrenia." Working with schizophrenic patients evokes a variety of painful emotions, such as guilt, fear, pity, anger, frustration, burnout, repulsion, and hopelessness. You'll need to acknowledge your feelings and acquire accurate information about these patients to guard against prejudices that may interfere with your care.

Emotional stress may cause you to avoid a patient, perhaps by rationalizing that he prefers isolation. But the patient you'd be most apt to avoid is often the one most likely to suffer from loneliness. Wishing to avoid him is normal—don't feel guilty about it. But you also mustn't allow your feelings to interfere with your professional responsibility. Ask the psychiatric liaison nurse or psychiatrist for help if your feelings interfere with forming a one-to-one relationship with the patient or making firm decisions about his care.

Also seek help from the liaison nurse, psychiatrist, or other members of the health care team if:
• you become concerned about your personal safety when dealing with an acutely psychotic or confused patient. Ask for help in evaluating the patient's potential for violent behavior. In addition, familiarize yourself with your hospital policy manual and follow outlined safety procedures.
• you start to identify with a patient who shares your age, interests, or experiences. Such feelings can become painful and interfere with your objectivity, even to the point where you fear becoming schizophrenic.
• you have difficulty dealing with the patient's dependency and fear of rejection. This is tricky; the patient may interpret your efforts to foster independence as rejection. He's also liable to feel hurt and angry when the therapeutic relationship comes to its end. You must acknowledge the patient's need to be dependent, while encouraging him to become independent.

stressors that trigger distorted perceptions. As a following step, you may explore the meaning of the patient's false beliefs.

Once thoughts become more organized and behavior improves, get the patient involved in occupational or recreational therapy. Focusing on reality-based activities will divert attention away from inward fantasies. Encourage the patient to develop skill in conceptual validation—gauging the accuracy of perceptions by comparing them with the views of others. For example, a patient may assume that people are laughing at him when in fact they're watching a television comedy. Encourage him to test this assumption by asking a member of the group to explain what's funny. You may also want to test the accuracy of your perceptions regarding the patient by comparing them to your perceptions of other patients and staff. This will help you judge aspects of care, such as the stage of trust in your relationship and the degree of dependency the patient requires.

Enlisting family support. Family involvement is important in all phases of treatment, from admission through discharge into a community or outpatient program. Find out what kinds of support family members need to continue coping with the patient. Depending on their needs, tell family members about the availability of financial aid and respite care. You may become instrumental in forming family education and support groups. These groups are especially helpful because most families are reluctant to express anger or guilt or to discuss mental illness with friends or relatives.

Shortened hospitalizations may also create difficulty for family members. Patients may return home while still exhibiting some schizophrenic symptoms. Help families cope with early discharge by teaching them to:
• recognize symptoms that suggest a need for medication adjustment or hospitalization
• cooperate in the patient's long-term treatment, for example, by giving medications and encouraging the patient to attend vocational training
• make use of community support systems and self-help groups such as the National Alliance for the Mentally Ill (NAMI)
• recognize what causes stress in the patient, and understand the effects of stress and how to manage it
• deal honestly with their own emotional distress regarding the patient.

Evaluation
Base your patient evaluation on the expected outcomes listed in your nursing care plan. To decide whether the patient's improved, ask yourself questions like these:
• Has the patient's anxiety level decreased?
• Does he still experience hallucinations?

The answers to these and other questions will help you assess your patient's mental status and the effectiveness of his care. Remember that the above questions are based on the sample nursing care plan found on page 99; your questions may differ.

Delusional Disorders: Fixed False Beliefs

Margaret Knowlton, a psychiatric clinical nurse specialist at Roger Williams General Hospital, Providence, R.I., wrote this chapter. She earned her BSN at Salve Regina College, Newport, R.I., and her MS from Boston University.

In a delusional disorder, a patient holds onto a belief that's false but not altogether implausible. The delusion doesn't result from any other mental disorder or from an organic cause and constitutes the patient's primary problem. The revised third edition of *Diagnostic and Statistical Manual of Mental Disorders* (DSM-III-R) establishes the following criteria for delusional disorders:

• The delusions are nonbizarre, involving situations that could be true. For example, the patient may believe somebody is following him or wants to poison him. Other delusions may focus on having a disease or deception by a spouse or lover.
• The delusions last for at least 1 month.
• The patient may have auditory or visual hallucinations, but these aren't prominent.
• Apart from the delusion and its ramifications, the patient doesn't behave strangely.

Until recently, delusional disorders were called paranoid disorders. However, DSM-III-R dropped the label "paranoid" because of its persecutory connotations. (See *What paranoia means.*) Delusions, though possibly involving persecution, may also involve erotomanic, grandiose, jealous, or somatic themes. In addition, they may have more than one theme. Unspecified delusions show no dominant theme. (See *Delusional themes.*)

Causes

The causes of delusional disorders remain unknown, but most theories focus on psychodynamic disturbances. (See *What causes delusional disorders?*, page 106.) Biochemical or neuropathologic changes apparently don't cause them. Although amphetamine use may cause paranoid psychosis, this effect can't be clearly explained as the result of norepinephrine or dopamine release or monoamine oxidase inhibition. What's more, genetic studies don't indicate a hereditary link. Women, though, succumb to the disorders more commonly than men.

Psychosocial factors. Psychosocial stress may play an important role in development of delusional disorders. The delusional patient probably has greater difficulty adjusting to loss, whether financial, social, emotional, physical, or intellectual.

Delusional disorders seem to strike most commonly between ages 35 and 55. Symptoms appear at a time when stress and responsibilities increase, opportunities wane, and the patient faces more and more disappointments and compromises.

Certain rare delusional disorders seem clearly related to psychosocial stress. For example, in induced psychotic disorder (*folie à deux*), the dominant person in a relationship transfers false beliefs to the partner. In migration psychosis, the patient experiences delusions probably caused by the stress associated with immigration.

Isolation born out of sensory deprivation may contribute to delusions. Paranoid symptoms, for instance, appear more frequently among deaf psychotics than among psychotics with normal hearing. To a lesser extent, blindness may be a factor. What's more, imprisonment, especially solitary confinement, may lead to paranoia (prison psychosis).

What paranoia means

Derived from the Greek words *para* (beside) and *nous* (mind), paranoia meant insanity in early Greek literature. Beginning in the 19th century, German psychiatrists who were studying delusions of persecution and grandeur revived the term. By the 1860s, it had come to mean chronic delusional conditions. In fact, an important 19th-century German psychiatry textbook defined paranoia as prolonged, systematic delusions (without predominant hallucinations) that do not lead to mental deterioration. Although this definition resembles modern day criteria for delusional disorders, common use of the word "paranoia" has become strongly associated with excessive suspiciousness or persecutory obsessions. As a result, the replacement of the label "paranoid disorders" with "delusional disorders" indicates an effort to correct the notion that paranoid delusions involve only persecutory themes.

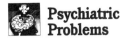
Delusional Disorders

Delusional themes

Common themes appear in delusions, ranging from erotomanic to somatic ones.

Erotomanic delusions

A prevalent delusional theme, erotomanic delusions concern romantic or spiritual love. The patient believes he shares in a idealized (rather than sexual) relationship with someone of higher status—a superior at work, a celebrity, or an anonymous stranger. The patient may hold this delusion in secret, but more commonly will try to contact the object of his delusion through calls, letters, gifts, or even spying. The patient may attempt to rescue his beloved from imagined danger. Patients with erotomanic delusions frequently harass public figures and often come to the attention of the police.

Grandiose delusions

The patient has a delusion that he has great, unrecognized talent, special insight, prophetic power, or has made an important discovery. To achieve recognition, he may contact government agencies, such as the Patent Office or the FBI. The patient with a religiously oriented delusion of grandeur may become a cult leader. Less commonly, he believes he shares a special relationship with some well-known personality, such as a rock-and-roll star or a world leader. The patient may believe himself to be a famous person, his identity usurped by an imposter.

Jealous delusions

These delusions focus on infidelity. For example, a patient may believe, without cause, that his lover has acted unfaithfully and may find evidence to justify the delusion, such as spots on bed sheets. He may confront his lover, try to control her movements, follow her, or track down her suspected paramour. He may physically attack her or, less likely, his perceived rival.

Persecutory delusions

The most common theme, the patient believes he's being followed, harassed, plotted against, poisoned, mocked, or deliberately prevented from achieving his long-term goals. He may perceive a simple or complex persecution scheme. If he develops a delusional system, he may interpret slight offenses as part of the scheme. If he perceives injustice, he may file numerous lawsuits or seek redress from government agencies (querulous paranoia). A patient who becomes resentful and angry may lash out violently against whoever he believes is hurting him.

Somatic delusions

The patient may perceive a foul odor coming from his skin, mouth, rectum, or other body part. Other delusions involve skin-crawling insects, internal parasites, and dysfunctional body parts.

Understanding delusional thinking. The delusional patient employs projection as a basic defense mechanism, attributing his own thoughts and feelings to others. He also mistrusts others, readily blames them, misinterprets their behavior, and rationalizes his own.

The patient's likely to feel insecure and suffer from low self-esteem and poor coping skills. If he's socially isolated, he may find coping with emptiness, anxiety, and loneliness to be especially painful. His increased dwelling on inner thoughts and dissatisfactions may worsen his anxiety. Narcissism, the belief that all events center on oneself, further clouds his understanding of the world and people around him. At first, the patient denies his painful feelings. But when denial no longer works, he develops delusional beliefs to project painful feelings onto others. As stress increases, the patient employs additional defense mechanisms, such as:

• reaction formation—repressing unacceptable feelings and reinforcing the opposite feelings. Reaction formation enables the patient to act with self-assurance and control when inwardly he feels powerless and dependent. He may believe he has a special gift for controlling or persuading others.

• rationalization—developing a well-reasoned explanation to justify delusional thinking.

• ideas of reference—fantasizing to the point where everything in the environment takes on a personal significance.

• creation of a delusional system—developing a well-organized group of beliefs, supported by a complex logical framework, to support the delusion.

• compartmentalization—keeping the delusion apart from other spheres of life. This enables the patient to appear normal.

Continued on page 106

Delusional Disorders

What causes delusional disorders?

Psychoanalysts from Freud to Fenichal have attempted to fathom the cause of delusional disorders.

Sigmund Freud, for instance, explained paranoia as a response to repressed homosexual wishes. According to Freud, the repressed desire ("I love him") emerged as the opposite ("I hate him") and through projection became a persecutory delusion ("He hates me"). The notion that paranoia results from repressed homosexual wishes has since fallen out of favor, but Freud's view has greatly influenced modern concepts of projection and reaction formation.

Harry Stack Sullivan proposed that the paranoid person's deep sense of inferiority, insecurity, and rejection cause unbearable feelings of loneliness and unworthiness. The paranoid gains a sense of security by projecting painful feelings onto others.

Melanie Klein focused on fixations that occur in early stages of childhood development to explain delusional thinking. The child projects aggressive impulses onto his mother and then incorporates the mother as an internal persecutor. Although many of Klein's views are controversial, her theory made an important contribution by moving away from the Freudian focus on the libido as the source of aggressive behavior.

Otto Fenichal emphasizes the role of the superego in paranoid delusions. A strict superego and unrealistic personal expectations cause internalization of guilt and feelings of inadequacy, which are projected in the form of sadistic delusions.

Continued

• paranoid resolution—completely transferring all insecurities and difficulties to the outside world. The patient becomes calm and secure in his delusion. (See *Dynamics of delusional thinking.*)

Recognizing pathologic suspicion. Nondelusional individuals become anxious or insecure when they perceive a threat to their interests, a perception that often has some basis in reality. They respond with an appropriate degree of sensitivity and vigilance and retain the ability to interpret events in a manner fairly consistent with the facts. Moreover, they do not respond to all situations with equal distrust.

In contrast, the delusional patient always reacts with hypersensitivity and extreme vigilance, constantly monitoring the environment for a hidden enemy. He anticipates threats and interprets events in a way that fits his delusion, ignoring any fact that doesn't fit. For example, he may claim the nursing staff is holding him captive. He may act on his false beliefs by telephoning the president of the hospital or a lawyer. Next, he may insist the nurse or doctor wants to poison him and refuse to eat. The patient will reject any rational arguments opposed to his delusion, though otherwise his thinking appears appropriate.

Assessment

Delusional patients often function well, aside from behavior related to their delusions. Their intellectual capabilities remain adequate and job performance continues satisfactorily. Their personalities usually remain well integrated in many areas. However, patients often suffer from poor social and marital relationships. In fact, about one third of them are widowed, divorced, or separated at the time of first admission.

Secretive, isolated, and with strong self-control, patients may live their lives without anyone discovering their illness. Sometimes, their delusions will become apparent to family or close friends during an emergency. At other times, discovery will occur during a routine physical examination, legal confrontation, employment examination, nursing admission assessment, or a chance personal encounter.

Assessing the patient accurately may prove difficult. He may deny feeling any distress and tell you he doesn't need help. If you ask why he was admitted to the hospital, he may reply that he needed a rest.

Observe for nonverbal cues indicating suspiciousness or mistrust; for example, upon entering a room, he may glance warily around and approach slowly. He may listen intently, looking for hidden meanings and becoming defensive upon hearing perceived insults. He may sit at the edge of his seat or fold his arms as if to shield himself. If he carries papers or money, he may clutch them firmly.

Be alert for signs of denial, projection, and rationalization. Once delusions become firmly entrenched, the patient will no longer seek to rationalize his beliefs. However, if he's still struggling to maintain his delusional defenses, he may make statements that reveal his condition, such as "People at work won't talk to me because I'm smarter than them" or "I have to lock up the refrigerator so the people next door won't steal my food."

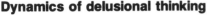
Delusional Disorders

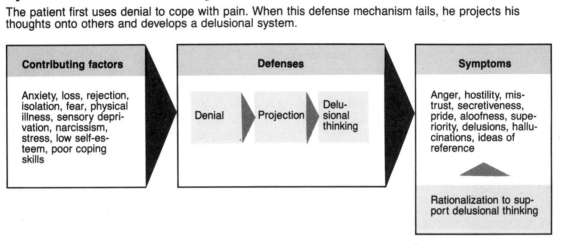

Dynamics of delusional thinking

The patient first uses denial to cope with pain. When this defense mechanism fails, he projects his thoughts onto others and develops a delusional system.

Contributing factors

Anxiety, loss, rejection, isolation, fear, physical illness, sensory deprivation, narcissism, stress, low self-esteem, poor coping skills

Defenses

Denial → Projection → Delusional thinking

Symptoms

Anger, hostility, mistrust, secretiveness, pride, aloofness, superiority, delusions, hallucinations, ideas of reference

Rationalization to support delusional thinking

Also be alert for accusatory statements. If the patient loses or forgets things, he might say, "Somebody keeps hiding my possessions" or "Nobody bothers to tell me anything." A patient who has been fired may say, "I lost my job because my boss is incompetent." A patient who is socially isolated may say, "No woman wants to date you if you're not a millionaire." Family members often regard the patient as chronically jealous or suspicious.

Note the patient's approach in presenting his history. The patient may speak with extreme reluctance, evaluating your intentions before revealing any information about himself. He may try to control the interview and appear superior to you, emphasizing what he has achieved, prominent people he knows, or places he has traveled.

The patient may become overly talkative, explaining events in great detail without making any clear points. Statements that first seem logical may later strike you as irrelevant. His circumstantial or hesitant speech may add to your confusion.

Information may seem contradictory, jumbled, or out of tune with reality. At the end of a long interview, you may remain confused about the patient's precise meaning. For example, you may not be able to tell whether the patient is being mistreated by a cruel landlord or a vindictive daughter-in-law.

Assess for signs of social isolation or hostility. Depressive symptoms and sexual problems frequently accompany the disorder. If asked about feeling lonely, angry, or defensive, the patient fervently denies these feelings. He may criticize others for their shortcomings or place unreasonable demands on friends and associates. However, he rarely acts violently. When hospitalized, he may have difficulty accepting his status as a patient, refusing to share a room and looking down upon other patients. At home, he may refuse to even open the door for a visiting nurse.

Be aware of your feelings during the interview. You may sense an emotional gap dividing you and the patient. If he's acting superior as a defense, you may feel slighted. If he projects his feelings of anxiety and insecurity onto you, you may feel belittled, blamed, or under attack. You may become caught in a confrontation with the

Continued on page 108

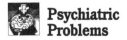 **Psychiatric Problems**

Delusional Disorders

Delusional symptoms in other conditions

Delusional symptoms also occur in such disorders as cognitive impairment, depression, drug and alcohol abuse, and paraphrenia.

Cognitive impairment

The patient who has reversible or irreversible cognitive impairment often exhibits the symptom of suspicion. When confronted with evidence of diminished function, he may become very indignant, making elaborate excuses and blaming others for his condition—usually close friends or family. The patient's thoughts seem unrealistic, poorly organized, and self-aggrandizing, and the theme of his suspicions may vary each day, making delusions easy to recognize.

Depression

In psychotic depression, the patient may be suspicious, even to the point of refusing help from well-meaning individuals. He may believe others seek to poison or persecute him, and you may have difficulty convincing him otherwise. The lower his self-esteem, the more likely the patient will suspect others.

Drug and alcohol abuse

Paranoid ideation commonly occurs with heavy alcohol consumption, alcohol withdrawal, amphetamine and marijuana use, chronic bromide intoxication, barbiturate and cocaine abuse, and withdrawal from barbiturates, minor tranquilizers, and hypnotic agents.

Paraphrenia

The patient with paraphrenia, a late-life schizophrenia, characteristically exhibits paranoid symptoms. The patient, most likely female, lives alone, suffers from partial deafness, and has few close relatives or associates. Regarded as eccentric, she appears to have an intact personality but adheres strongly to well-organized delusions. Vivid, threatening hallucinations may occur. In response to disturbed perceptions, the patient may run away or commit suicide. The patient may improve following treatment with phenothiazines, but will continue to lack insight into her condition and probably never understand that her paranoid beliefs were delusional.

Continued

patient or find yourself becoming guarded, pulling back, or wanting to retaliate.

Differential diagnosis. Conclusively diagnosing delusional disorders requires ruling out other emotional or organic causes of delusion. Use of alcohol, amphetamines, cocaine and other drugs, dementia, and infectious, metabolic, and endocrine disorders may all lead to delusion symptoms. A thorough health history, physical assessment, and routine laboratory tests will help rule out an organic disorder.

You may have difficulty differentiating delusional disorder from schizophrenia or mood disorders. Remember the following:
• Schizophrenics experience bizarre delusions and prominent hallucinations, but patients with delusional disorders experience non-bizarre delusions and rarely have prominent hallucinations.
• Paranoid schizophrenics have symptoms of schizophrenia along with paranoid characteristics. Delusional patients do not develop schizophrenic symptoms, such as disorganized behavior.
• Delusional patients don't develop full depressive or manic syndromes. Mood disturbances usually develop after delusions and last briefly. (See *Delusional symptoms in other conditions.*)

Planning

When planning care for the delusional patient, focus on his suspicious behavior and perception of reality. Assess the patient's readiness to listen and to accept objective feedback on his condition. Before you prepare the plan, develop the nursing diagnosis by identifying the patient's problem or potential problem and relating it to its cause. Possible nursing diagnoses include:
• anxiety; related to mistrust
• coping, ineffective individual; related to fear of exploitation by family and friends
• fear; related to perception of a conspiracy
• nutrition, altered (less than body requirements); related to belief that food is poisoned
• social interaction, impaired; related to mistrust
• social isolation; related to fear of being misunderstood
• thought processes, altered; related to inability to validate reality.

The sample nursing care plan on the opposite page shows expected outcomes, nursing interventions, and discharge planning for one nursing diagnosis. You'll want to individualize your care plan to meet the needs of your patient and his family.

Intervention

Usually, psychotherapy and drug therapy together work best. The patient probably will not require inpatient treatment unless his behavior becomes dangerous to himself or others. Involuntary hospitalization can reinforce the patient's suspiciousness and hinder compliance.

Because of the patient's mistrust, hypersensitivity, and tendency to misinterpret others, he may not benefit from group or insight-oriented psychotherapy. Psychotherapists usually tailor psychosocial treatment according to the patient's needs. After establishing

Delusional Disorders

Sample nursing care plan: Delusional disorder

Nursing diagnosis	Expected outcomes
Anxiety; related to mistrust	The patient will: • cooperate with treatment. • not report feeling coerced by staff. • communicate a sense of receiving more understanding from others.

Nursing interventions	Discharge planning
• Determine extent of the patient's mistrust. • Allow him to express his concerns. • Emphasize reality gently, without argument, to the patient. • Give him accurate and concise information before administering medications or treatments. • Allow him to make choices to give a measure of control over his care, when possible.	• Arrange follow-up appointments with the therapist or community mental health clinic. • Provide written instructions for taking medications, including schedule and possible adverse reactions, when appropriate. • Teach patient, family, and friends early signs of relapse, such as increased anxiety, suspiciousness, and sleep disturbances.

a therapeutic relationship, the psychotherapist may then gently challenge the patient's delusional beliefs.

Neuroleptic drugs help treat the disorder and accompanying anxiety, agitation, and psychotic symptoms. Commonly used drugs include chlorpromazine (Thorazine), thioridazine (Mellaril), trifluoperazine (Stelazine), or haloperidol (Haldol). If the patient suspects poisoning, he may refuse oral drug administration. Such patients may benefit from periodic injections.

Certain other treatments, used in the past, have now fallen out of favor. These include electroconvulsive therapy, insulin shock therapy, and psychosurgery.

Nursing care measures. Paranoid beliefs indicate poor communication, alienation, and lack of trust. As a result, you'll need to initially establish clear and honest communication with the patient. Direct your efforts toward reassuring him and encouraging compliance with prescribed treatment. Consider suggesting that he seek treatment for depression or anxiety before even mentioning his delusional beliefs. Later, when dealing with delusions, don't condemn or agree with them. Instead, gently show the patient how they interfere with his life.

Don't mix medication with food in an effort to force compliance. Serve food in closed containers if the patient fears poisoning.

If the patient becomes hostile or angry, remember always that fear and anxiety underlie his reaction. (See *When a delusional patient becomes angry,* page 110.) You may need to consult with a psychiatric liaison nurse or a psychiatrist to explore your own feelings. Be especially prepared for hostility if the patient entered the hospital for medical illness or surgery or because of other circumstances beyond his control.

Maintain a respectful distance from the patient. Displaying too much warmth may frighten him and cause him to suspect your motives.

If the patient has family or friends, consider asking his permission to include them in treatment. This may decrease his sense of isolation. Find out if he has been in psychotherapy and ask whether he'd like to include his therapist in his care during hospitalization.

Continued on page 110

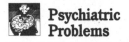
Delusional Disorders

When a delusional patient becomes angry

When caring for a delusional patient, prepare yourself to deal effectively with his anger. By acting appropriately, you can calm him and help him cope. However, ill-considered actions may exacerbate angry and hostile feelings.

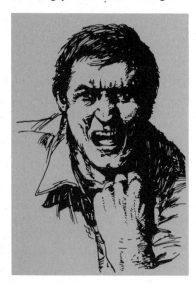

Consider the following guidelines:
• Remain calm and speak softly.
• Address the patient by name.
• Closely observe his body language and monitor your own for signs of hostility; keep your stance relaxed and as neutral as possible.
• When listening to his complaints, give undivided attention and maintain eye contact.
• Restate his remarks to try and identify his real concern.
• Demonstrate your concern for his welfare by explaining your intended actions.
• Don't promise what you can't deliver.
• Explain your limitations in resolving a problem, and call for help if the situation is beyond your authority or control.

Continued

Evaluation

Base your evaluation on the expected outcomes listed in the nursing care plan. To determine if the patient has improved, ask yourself questions like these:
• Does the patient cooperate with treatment?
• Has he mentioned coercion by the staff?
• Has he stated that he's feeling more secure and better understood?

Your answers to these questions will help you evaluate your patient's status and the effectiveness of his care. Keep in mind that these questions are based on the sample care plan shown on page 109. Your questions may differ.

Self-test

1. Characteristics of positive schizophrenia include all of the following except:
a. hallucinations **b.** inability to experience pleasure **c.** bizarre behavior **d.** thought disorders

2. Hallucinations constitute the only definitive symptom of schizophrenia.
a. true **b.** false

3. Which of the following statements about neuroleptic drugs is false?
a. Their actions provide the basis for the dopamine hypothesis.
b. They act most effectively during the late stages of the patient's illness. **c.** They can cause irreversible neurologic damage. **d.** Their successful use hasn't eliminated the need for psychosocial interventions.

4. Patients with delusional disorders characteristically exhibit all the following symptoms except:
a. ideas of reference **b.** preservation of intellectual capabilities
c. full depressive or manic episodes **d.** denial of feelings

5. All of the following are recommended interventions for delusional disorders except:
a. Suggest that the patient seek help for anxiety or depression without referring to his delusional beliefs. **b.** Gently explain how delusions interfere with his life. **c.** Explain your own limitations if you can't meet his demands. **d.** If the patient refuses to take prescribed medication, mix it with his food.

Answers (page numbers show where answer appears in text)
1. **b** (page 91) 2. **b** (page 99) 3. **b** (page 100) 4. **c** (page 108)
5. **d** (page 109)

Substance Abuse and Eating Disorders: Alcohol, Drug, and Food Abuse

Sarah L. Mynatt, an associate professor at the Memphis State University School of Nursing, co-wrote this chapter. She earned her BSN and MS from the University of Tennessee College of Nursing and her EdD from Memphis State University.

Co-author **Margaret Marx Aiken** is an assistant professor at Memphis State University School of Nursing. She earned her BA from Manhattanville College, Purchase, N.Y., and her MSN from the University of Texas at Austin School of Nursing.

Perhaps one of your greatest challenges in dealing with substance abuse patients will be preventing your own feelings from interfering with assessment and treatment. Although many of these patients will manipulate, deceive, and commit crimes to obtain drugs or alcohol, you'll need to avoid frowning on their behavior. Their complex illness can best be treated in an objective way, without overtones of moral failings and reproach.

When caring for patients with eating disorders, you'll face a somewhat different challenge. Affected patients, primarily women, require help in overcoming psychological obstacles to healthful eating. Some may even require life-sustaining feedings, such as total parenteral nutrition.

Substance abuse

Substance abuse refers to regular use of alcohol or a drug that affects the central nervous system and causes behavioral changes. It follows a pathologic course, impairs social or job function, and lasts at least 1 month. It may lead to dependency, in which the patient can't control use of the substance and develops withdrawal symptoms if he attempts to stop or reduce intake. (See *Vocabulary of abuse*, page 112.)

Substance abusers share key personality traits. Although outwardly dominant and critical of others, they're inwardly passive and full of self-doubt. They're described by psychologists as being fixated early in their psychosexual development. They often have problems with sexual identification and may act promiscuously, dress inappropriately, and have trouble forming intimate relationships. Rebellious and narcissistic, they use defense mechanisms such as escapism, denial, and rationalization to justify their behavior. (See *Profile of the chemically dependent patient*, page 112.)

In addition to psychological makeup, numerous social, environmental, and biological influences may cause an individual to turn to drugs and alcohol. A slum dweller may seek to escape feelings of hopelessness and defeat. Members of the upper-middle class may seek to escape from intense social, financial, or academic pressure. Teenagers may seek to ease feelings of alienation and powerlessness or to conform to peer pressure.

Heredity appears to strongly influence an individual's likelihood of becoming an alcoholic. What's more, an environment that provides easy access to alcohol or drugs will increase the likelihood of abuse. Occupational stress also plays a part in chemical dependency. Nurses, for example, have a dependency rate 50% higher than the general population.

But whatever initiates drug or alcohol use, the individual must obtain pleasure from the substance for his habit to continue. He may find that drugs or alcohol help him to relax, alleviate boredom, ease painful emotions, escape from reality, enhance perception, or experience mystical or religious insights. Over time, his dependence increases as he becomes caught in a pattern of compulsive drug seeking and loses control over drug use and his life.

Continued on page 112

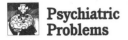
Substance Abuse and Eating Disorders

Profile of the chemically dependent patient

Chemically dependent patients may exhibit certain key personality traits and behavior patterns. When assessing a chemically dependent patient, note if he:
• suffers from low self-esteem and lack of ego strength
• has trouble conforming socially despite a strong need to belong
• feels anxious, depressed, and guilty
• behaves inconsistently and impulsively and manipulates others
• seeks short-term gratification
• lies about the quantity of drug or alcohol ingested
• hides drug or alcohol supply
• becomes isolated socially
• fears rejection
• acquires new friends who also use drugs or alcohol and abandons old friends who don't
• experiences blackouts
• develops increased tolerance
• loses control over chemical use
• denies a chemical dependency problem
• rationalizes to defend irresponsible or self-destructive behavior
• projects feelings of guilt, inadequacy, and low self-esteem onto a family member
• arrives at work late, leaves early, or frequently misses work altogther
• misses work deadlines or becomes less productive
• stops participating in preventive health activities
• loses control over life, with all activities directed toward satisfying the drug or alcohol habit
• frequently experiences work-related accidents
• frequently enters hospital for problems associated with chemical dependency.

When working with a chemically dependent adolescent, take note if he:
• dislikes school
• associates with peers who use alcohol or drugs
• fears failure
• feels curious about effects of alcohol and drugs
• has difficulty dealing with unpleasant emotions
• rebels against family authority
• has a poor relationship with his parents.

Vocabulary of abuse

By reviewing the definitions below, you'll become familiar with the terms commonly used in discussions of substance abuse.

Addiction
Physical dependence on a drug. Because a drug alters the patient's physiology, withdrawal causes moderate to life-threatening symptoms.

Chemical dependence
Psychological or physical dependence, or both, following continual or occasional drug use.

Cross-tolerance
Property that allows one drug to be substituted for another without a loss of tolerance.

Drug abuse
Intake of prescribed or nonprescribed drugs unrelated to a specific health problem and outside of a generally accepted medical context.

Drug use
Ingestion of any chemical substance that affects the body, including illegal, legal, and medically prescribed drugs.

Habituation
Dependence on a drug to provide pleasure, relief from stress, or other psychological benefits. This dependence outweighs consideration of possible adverse consequences of drug use, such as family problems and job loss.

Substance abuse
Extreme or unhealthful use of alcohol, tobacco, drugs, or food. Substance abuse may be chronic or episodic.

Substance dependence
A form of substance abuse characterized by psychological or physiologic dependence, or both, as evidenced by tolerance or withdrawal. Other terms for dependence include addiction and habituation.

Tolerance
A mechanism by which the brain adjusts to repeated doses of a drug, requiring the user to increase dosage to produce the desired effect.

Withdrawal
Symptoms that develop when a chemically dependent patient curtails or stops drug use. Withdrawal symptoms vary, depending on the abused substance.

Substance abuse—*continued*

Chemical dependency causes irreparable damage to the body's organs and tissues. Like other chronic diseases, it's distinguished by periods of remission and exacerbation. Like other progressive diseases, it follows a predictable course. (See *Three phases of addiction*.)

Finally, chemical dependency can't be cured. For example, only if an alcoholic abstains from drinking will he be able to lead a normal life. If he takes even one drink, he'll risk returning to a debilitated condition, the same as if he never stopped drinking.

Assessment

Your approach will depend on the patient's condition. If the patient suffers from such complications as alcohol withdrawal delerium (commonly known as delerium tremens), hepatic coma, esophageal varices, respiratory depression, gastric bleeding, or dysrhythmias, treat these problems first. Afterward, you can address the chemical dependency.

Substance Abuse and Eating Disorders

Three phases of addiction

1

In the *progressive or early phase*, the person addicted to drugs or alcohol:
• denies addiction
• sneaks alcohol or drugs
• experiences blackouts
• uses alcohol or drugs to cope
• becomes angry easily
• lies to cover up habit
• avoids references to alcohol or drugs
• develops increased tolerance
• begins to lose control.

2

In the *crucial phase*, the addict:
• justifies behavior
• feels angry and guilty
• develops paranoid traits
• behaves extravagantly
• changes pattern of alcohol or drug use
• encounters job and marital problems
• maintains a constant supply of alcohol or drugs
• develops physical and psychological problems
• swears off alcohol or drugs
• experiences indefinable fears
• loses friends.

3

In the *chronic phase*, the addict:
• experiences tremors
• deteriorates physically and psychologically
• becomes divorced
• spends time in jail
• suffers serious financial setbacks
• loses job
• experiences breakdown of value system
• faces collapse of support system.

If the patient is obviously intoxicated or high, keep your questions simple and to the point. Ask when was his last drink and what drugs he has taken in the last 24 hours and in the last week. Then ask about symptoms. Try to establish rapport quickly. If friends or relatives have accompanied the patient to the hospital, ask them for relevant information. Also study any previous medical records. The patient may have to be examined for an accompanying condition, such as hypertension, diabetes, or a seizure disorder. If the patient appears coherent, seek more detailed information on his pattern of abuse. (See *Assessing chemically dependent patients*, page 114.)

Physical examination. Substance abuse affects every organ and body system. While many symptoms are specific to particular substances, common indicators of abuse do exist. When assessing for any kind of substance abuse, form an impression of the patient's general appearance. Note if the patient seems unkempt, nervous, or agitated. Does he pace around the room? Does he show signs of tremors? Ask the patient if he's had difficulty sleeping. Also take his vital signs, being alert for increased blood pressure (common in alcohol intoxication and withdrawal).

Central nervous system (CNS). Assess for alertness, coherence, and orientation to time, person, and place. Does the patient walk with an unsteady or awkward gait? You may perform the Romberg test to assess for cerebellar dysfunction. To perform the test, have the patient stand erect with his feet together and his arms at his sides. Ask him to hold this position with his eyes open, then closed. In cerebellar dysfunction, the patient will have difficulty keeping his balance.

Head and neck. Check for lesions or injuries, head lice (common in some juveniles and in homeless or indigent patients), distended neck veins, petechiae on the nose and cheeks, and ruddy complexion. Observe the sclera of his eyes for redness or yellowing. Test pupillary response.

Chest. Assess for irregular heart rate and rhythm, wheezing, abnormal breath sounds (such as crackles or rhonchi), and symptoms of obstructive pulmonary disease. Patients who smoke marijuana regularly or freebase cocaine commonly have difficulty breathing. Cocaine freebasers may feel as if their hearts are racing.

Abdomen. Observe for ascites, distended or tender abdomen, and enlarged liver or spleen. If the liver appears large, assess for ecchymoses or other signs of bleeding. The patient may spit up blood or have dark, foul, tarry stools.

Skin. Observe for spider hemangiomas, yellowed skin (a sign of liver damage), bruised or edematous legs, poor skin turgor in the legs, weak pedal pulses, and loss of muscle mass.

Nutritional status. The chemically dependent patient usually doesn't eat regularly and may become severely malnourished. Ask the patient what he usually eats, if he's experienced recent weight changes, what he considers a balanced diet, whether he cooks for himself, and whether he takes vitamin supplements. Alcoholics need more vitamin B complex because alcohol interferes with vitamin B me-

Continued on page 114

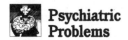
Substance Abuse and Eating Disorders

Assessing chemically dependent patients

Ask these questions during your interview with chemically dependent patients.

☐ What drugs, including alcohol, do you regularly take?
☐ How often and how much do you take?
☐ When did you last use drugs or alcohol?
☐ How long have you been using drugs or drinking?
☐ When was the first time you used drugs or alcohol, and how did you react?
☐ Do any relatives have a history of alcohol or drug abuse? (If so, this could make the patient's recovery more difficult.)
☐ What drugs have you tried? (To refresh the patient's memory, show him a list of drugs and ask him to answer yes or no.)

Whenever the patient admits to using a particular drug, ask him specific questions about his pattern of use—when, how much, how long, and the effects.

Looking at the patient's family

While the dependent person is under the influence of alcohol or drugs, his family is under his influence, caught in a complicated web of emotions—irritation, nervousness, guilt, shame, hurt, depression, and anger. On top of all this, they often feel lonely, not knowing where to turn for help.

Family members often unwittingly enable the chemically dependent person to follow an addictive lifestyle. One family member, usually the spouse, generally assumes the role of *primary enabler,* allowing the dependent person to continue his behavior or to even become worse. The enabler keeps everything in the family "going." Over time, the family may develop a high tolerance for bizarre behavior. Keep in mind that once the dependent person enters treatment, family members also need professional help to restore balance to their lives.

Substance abuse—*continued*

tabolism. If the patient is homeless, ask if he can obtain regular meals at a shelter.

Emotional assessment. Note any indications of depression, excitation, suicidal ideation, suspiciousness, anger, or anxiety. Observe for signs of instability, mood swings, unreasonable resentments, remorse, grandiosity, self-pity, and pathologic jealousy. Ask the patient if he's experienced hallucinations, memory loss, or problems with communication, following directions, finishing work, or controlling violent impulses. Also ask if he's ever received treatment for emotional problems. If so, determine the type and effectiveness of treatment.

Motivation. Ask why the patient decided to seek treatment. Did his family or employer insist? Did the courts require him to enter a treatment program? Or did he enter treatment seeking relief from symptoms caused by abuse? If he entered the hospital on his own, verify who he wants informed about his admission. Because of social stigma, many patients don't want others to know they're being treated.

Social support. Find out about social and family support to help you plan for the patient's treatment and discharge. If the patient identifies certain people as especially supportive, involve them in his treatment and ask them to help in his recovery after discharge. (See *Looking at the patient's family*.)

Diagnostic tests. Blood and urine analysis may detect the presence of alcohol or drugs. Standard blood tests include complete blood count with differential, prothrombin time, serum electrolytes and lipids, liver and renal function studies, fasting blood glucose, albumin with total protein, hepatitis B surface antigen, and serum B_{12} and folic acid levels. Other standard tests include stool guiac, urinalysis, chest X-ray, and EKG. The doctor may also order a computed tomography scan, a GI series, and an EEG.

Planning

Before writing your care plan, develop the nursing diagnosis by identifying the patient's problem or potential problem, then relating it to its cause. Possible nursing diagnoses for a chemically dependent patient include:
● injury, potential for; related to disorientation, tremors, or impaired judgment
● self-concept, disturbance in; related to guilt, mistrust, or ambivalence
● violence, potential for; related to emotional immaturity, high anxiety, or impulsive behavior
● nutrition, altered (less than body requirements); related to anorexia
● fluid volume deficit, potential for; related to abnormal fluid loss secondary to vomiting and diarrhea associated with withdrawal
● sleep pattern disturbance; related to irritability, tremors, and nightmares
● sexual dysfunction; related to impotence
● coping, ineffective individual; related to inability to manage stressors without drugs or alcohol

Substance Abuse and Eating Disorders

Sample nursing care plan: Chemical abuse

Nursing diagnosis	Expected outcomes
Sleep pattern disturbance; related to irritability, tremors, and nightmares	The patient will: • implement measures to promote sleep. • report a restful night's sleep.
Nursing interventions • Monitor patient's sleep patterns. • Explain the relationship between sleep and chemical abuse (for example, use of depressants may suppress REM sleep and use of cocaine may deplete amino acids in the brain). • Allow patient to express his feelings about sleep disturbance. • Encourage patient to participate in regular schedule of activities. • Check for adverse effects after giving medications. • Encourage quiet activities before bedtime.	**Discharge planning** • Consult with the psychiatric nurse specialist or community health nurse to provide follow-up home care, as needed. • Review with the patient and family the dynamics of sleep and chemical abuse. • Encourage the patient and his family to attend self-help groups, such as Alcoholics Anonymous, Alanon, or Narcotics Anonymous. • Advise the patient to socialize with people who don't abuse drugs or alcohol.

• social isolation; related to loss of work or withdrawal from others
• family processes, altered; related to disruption in marriage and inconsistent limit-setting.

The sample nursing care plan above shows expected outcomes, nursing interventions, and discharge planning for one nursing diagnosis listed above. Of course, you'll want to individualize your care plan to meet your patient's needs.

Intervention

In acute drug intoxication, treatment is symptomatic and depends upon the drug ingested. Interventions may include fluid replacement, nutritional and vitamin supplements, controlled and gradual withdrawal, sedatives to induce sleep, antidiarrheal agents to reduce GI distress, and symptomatic treatment of complications.

Meeting the patient's long-term needs, however, requires aggressive treatment of emotional problems as well as medical complications. Planning requires a careful evaluation and identification of any coexisting psychiatric problems.

Various treatment options exist. Patients may receive inpatient care or enter into drug-and-alcohol treatment facilities. Other patients attend outpatient, partial hospitalization, or residential programs. Some patients graduate to residential or outpatient programs after receiving inpatient care. Programs frequently combine education with individual, group, or family counseling, and often require participation in a support group, such as Alcoholics Anonymous (AA) or Narcotics Anonymous (NA).

The support that alcoholics and drug addicts receive at AA and NA meetings is vital to avoiding relapse. Open to all who seek help, AA and NA participants follow a 12-step program that insists upon total abstinence. AA, NA, and other anonymous groups share a common philosophy: they encourage the patient to take one day at a time, to accept his powerlessness over addiction, and to rely

Continued on page 116

Substance Abuse and Eating Disorders

Twelve steps of Alcoholics Anonymous

The chart below depicts the 12 steps of Alcoholics Anonymous. These steps offer a guideline for individuals struggling toward sobriety. Other anonymous groups, such as Narcotics Anonymous, use a similar program.

We admitted we were powerless over alcohol—that our lives had become unmanageable.

We came to believe that a Power greater than ourselves could restore us to sanity.

We made a decision to turn our will and our lives over to the care of God, as we understood Him.

We made a searching and fearless moral inventory of ourselves.

We made a list of all persons we had harmed, and became willing to make amends to them all.

We humbly asked Him to remove our shortcomings.

We were entirely ready to have God remove all these defects of character.

We admitted to God, to ourselves, and to another human being the exact nature of our wrongs.

We made direct amends to such people wherever possible, except when to do so would injure them or others.

We continued to take personal inventory and when we were wrong promptly admitted it.

We sought through prayer and meditation to improve our conscious contact with God, as we understood Him, praying only for knowledge of His will for us and the power to carry that out.

Having had a spiritual awakening as the result of these steps, we tried to carry this message to alcoholics, and to practice these principles in all our affairs.

Reprinted with permission of Alcoholics Anonymous World Services, Inc.

Dual diagnosis

Young urban-dwelling adults who suffer from both chronic mental illness and chemical dependency constitute a new population of the mentally ill. Evidence indicates that many first used drugs in an attempt to control symptoms of mental illness.

Many of these people go undiagnosed and untreated; others are diagnosed as having bipolar disorder, schizophrenia, or antisocial or borderline personality disorder but fail to comply with treatment.

Detoxifying and rehabilitating these patients is difficult. Before they can successfully undergo treatment for mental illness, they must free themselves from chemical dependency.

Substance abuse—*continued*

ultimately upon the power of God for freedom from addiction. (See *Twelve steps of Alcoholics Anonymous.*)

Psychiatric facilities. Psychological tests may indicate that a psychiatric disorder other than chemical dependency constitutes the patient's primary problem. For example, two thirds of alcoholics also suffer from depression, anxiety disorders, or attention deficit disorders. Such patients may be referred for treatment in a hospital psychiatric unit or psychiatric hospital. Patients with depression and other primary psychiatric disorders usually receive long-term therapy with psychotropic drugs. Alcoholics with secondary psychiatric symptoms may also receive drugs on a short-term basis. Note that using drug therapy for these patients conflicts with the AA philosophy, which prohibits the use of chemicals in recovery. (See *Dual diagnosis.*)

Nursing care measures. Your responsibilities will vary depending on the treatment setting, but may include:

• *Confronting the patient.* You may have to help other members of the treatment team break down the patient's denial of his dependency. This may mean challenging him with evidence of his de-

Substance Abuse and Eating Disorders

Developing self-awareness

To give effective, compassionate care to the chemically dependent patient, you must first examine your own feelings about addiction. This scrutinizing process includes:
• identifying your own attitudes and prejudices about alcohol and drug abuse
• identifying any past experiences that caused you to form negative attitudes toward alcoholics or drug abusers
• recognizing any personal weaknesses regarding the use of certain drugs or alcohol that might blind you to this problem in other people
• examining how you communicate with alcoholics and drug abusers, checking for judgmental, moralistic, or patronizing comments
• recognizing any tendency to avoid alcoholics and drug abusers

• identifying any tendency to take on a destructive role, such as persecutor (being judgmental or punitive), victim (allowing the patient to blame, use, or manipulate you), or enabler (accepting responsibility for the patient's behavior).

Once you've become aware of your feelings, acknowledge your limitations and seek appropriate assistance when caring for patients. Enlist the help of a psychiatric liaison nurse or psychiatrist, if necessary. Work to develop a positive attitude about helping the chemically dependent patient. Keep in mind the following points:
• Complicated and poorly understood, chemical dependency causes suffering for both the patient and his family.

• Chemically dependent people deserve the same respect and caring given to other patients.
• You can respect and help a patient without condoning or promoting self-destructive behavior.
• Chemical dependency can be prevented and treated, especially if it's recognized and acted on early.

If you deal honestly and objectively with the chemically dependent patient and his family, you won't have to feel personally responsible if he fails to kick his habit. Don't expect complete success—relapses occur, no matter what you do or how hard you try. This may not be your patient's first attempt to kick drugs or alcohol, so give him encouragement and emphasize his progress.

pendency. When doing so, remain calm and state the facts about chemical abuse and its consequences. Make it clear that you'll support him if he seeks treatment. Family members, friends, and employers may also try to get the patient to face up to his behavior and to obtain treatment.

• *Discussing the patient's responsibility for his own care.* Stress that the patient needs to participate in all therapeutic activities and cooperate with the staff if he wants to recover. Reassure him that staff members will provide support.

• *Supervising malnourished patients during meals.* Patients who can't maintain minimum nutrition may need to be fed parenterally.

• *Monitoring surgical patients.* Because of their poor nutrition and health, alcoholics and drug addicts make poor surgical risks. After surgery, observe the patient closely for nervousness, restlessness, and fearfulness, and notify the doctor immediately so he can start seizure precautions. These symptoms can worsen, resulting in delirium, seizures, and even death.

• *Providing education and counseling.* You may meet with individuals, groups, and families to discuss substance abuse. Topics may include developing new coping skills and making life-style changes. Some nurses use videotapes to initiate the discussion; others ask recovering alcoholics or drug addicts to speak. Patients often have serious occupational, health, family, and legal difficulties, and you'll have to collaborate with other members of the treatment team to help them to cope. To sharpen your skills, some facilities encourage nurses to attend support groups. For example, attending Alanon, a support group for families of alcoholics, may help in interacting effectively with the recovering alcoholics and their families. (See *Developing self-awareness.*)

Continued on page 118

Substance Abuse and Eating Disorders

Recognizing the nurse addict

High job stress combined with easy accessibility to drugs makes health care professionals, including nurses, especially susceptible to chemical abuse. Studies estimate that 10% to 20% of health care workers become chemically dependent.

Usually from a stable family background, the average chemically dependent nurse obtains her supply from a doctor, hospital, or pharmacy. She doesn't have a history of delinquency or adolescent drug or alcohol problems. Typically, she uses drugs or alcohol for pain, fatigue, or depression at first. An ambitious worker, she feels responsible toward her job and often continues to do excellent work until her dependency makes it impossible.

In addition, the chemically dependent nurse generally:
• uses drugs or alcohol alone
• rates high on impulse control on psychological tests
• has conventional values and attitudes
• ignores or denies feelings of depression, tension, boredom, or unhappiness
• feels guilty about her dependency.

Assessment

Increasingly, nurses are becoming aware of the need to help chemically dependent colleagues. The following outline lists some common warning signs that may alert you to chemical dependence in a colleague.

Behavioral signs. Look for irritability, argumentativeness, mood swings, increasing isolation, inappropriate responses, unkempt appearance, forgetfulness or memory lapses, confusion, decreased alertness, or euphoria. Problems may develop with her children or spouse. She may break down on the job.

Physical changes. Observe for flushed face, red eyes, unsteady gait, and slurred or accelerated speech. Her breath may smell of alcohol and her arms or fingers may show blisters, needle tracks, or burns from cigarettes. She may experience tremors, restlessness, diaphoresis, and pupillary changes. She may have a runny nose with flu-like symptoms. What's more, she may complain of headache, backache, or other vague aches and pains.

Signs of drug pilfering. Such signs include poor documentation and constant volunteering to give medications, count narcotics, or "float" to units that regularly administer pain medication. The chemically dependent nurse may arrive at work early, stay late, and frequently disappear throughout the shift. Her patients may complain of not getting pain relief (analgesics in vials may be replaced with water) or of not getting medication.

Changes in job performance. Such changes include absenteeism, poor work quality, and failure to meet deadlines. Charting may become illogical or sloppy and documentation may be inadequate.

Interventions

Although one might think that nurses would recover quickly from their addiction, they typically require more extensive treatment than other patients. After all, staying sober often requires a drastic change in life-style that makes it possible to avoid the people, places, and situations associated with drugs or alcohol. For most health care professionals, this would mean giving up a career.

Many rehabilitation facilities have developed long-term programs specifically for health care professionals. These programs may include inpatient treatment, outpatient treatment, supervised independent living, and a gradual return to work in partnership with another recovering health care professional. Most range in length from 6 months to a year or more, and many have proven successful in helping these individuals return to community life and to work.

Substance abuse—*continued*

Evaluation

Base your evaluation on the expected outcomes listed in the sample nursing care plan. To determine if the patient's improved, ask yourself questions like these:
• Does the patient participate in activities that promote sleep?
• Does he report having a peaceful night's sleep and feeling rested in the morning?

The answers to these and other questions will help you assess your patient's status and the effectiveness of his care. Keep in mind that these questions stem from the sample care plan on page 115. Your questions may differ.

Frequently abused substances

Alcohol

The National Institute of Alcohol Abuse estimates that 10% of the United States population is alcohol dependent. Government sources further estimate that 200,000 alcohol-related deaths occur each

Substance Abuse and Eating Disorders

What makes an alcoholic?
Biological, cultural, and social factors distinguish the alcoholic from the social drinker.

Biological factors
Heredity influences the predisposition to alcoholism more than any combination of social or environmental factors. For example, 95% of alcoholics have at least one relative with a drinking problem.

Research also indicates a biochemical basis for alcoholism. When an individual predisposed to alcoholism drinks, his body manufactures tetrahydroisoquinoline (TIQ), a product of heroin metabolism that's more addictive than morphine. The same process doesn't occur with social drinkers. Animal studies indicate that TIQ, once injected, remains permanently, which may explain why alcoholics can't become social drinkers even after remaining sober for a number of years.

Cultural factors
An individual's cultural background may greatly influence his vulnerability to alcoholism. For example, Mediterranean peoples and Jews have a low incidence of alcoholism, probably the result of having used alcohol in nondestructive ways over many generations. On the other hand, cultures more recently exposed to alcohol, such as American Indians and Australian Aborigines, have a high incidence of alcoholism.

Social factors
Difficult social or family relationships may cause an individual to turn to alcohol. People from broken homes, homes with an absent or rejecting father, or homes with a history of alcohol abuse are more apt to become alcoholic. People from teetotaler families face a high risk, possibly because family members have no experience in dealing with alcohol responsibly.

year. Other research indicates that death rates for alcoholics may be three times higher than that of the general population.

Because alcohol is widely available, legal, socially accepted, and affordable, it's all the more dangerous for individuals prone to chemical dependency. (See *What makes an alcoholic?* and *Alcoholism among women and the elderly,* page 120.)

A CNS depressant with sedative-anesthetic effects, alcohol is broken down primarily by the liver. Drinking alcohol may provide relief from anxiety. However, after drinking excessively to relieve anxiety, an individual may develop a hangover, accompanied by even more painful feelings of anxiety. Hangover symptoms may include malaise, nausea, vomiting, sweating, thirst, and flushing.

Other effects of alcohol use include:
- slowed brain function. Even with consumption of small amounts, alcohol may lead to impaired judgment, alertness, coordination, and reflexes.
- attitude and behavioral changes. The patient may become hostile or aggressive or take life-threatening risks.
- blackouts. Patients who drink heavily may experience anterograde amnesia—a loss of short-term memory with retention of remote memory, possibly caused by dehydration of brain tissue. The patient may function effectively during a blackout, yet have no memory of his activity. As alcoholism progresses, blackouts may indicate advanced physical dependence and may not have anything to do with how much the patient drinks.
- medical complications. Heavy, chronic users of alcohol face an increased risk of cirrhosis, gastritis, ulcers, pancreatitis, cardiomyopathy, anemia, peripheral neuropathy, sexual dysfunction, and cancer. Drinking during pregnancy may lead to fetal alcohol syndrome, the leading cause of mental retardation. Chronic alcohol abuse may also lead to such organic mental disorders as Wernicke's encephalopathy, characterized by truncal ataxia and confusion. Wernicke's encephalopathy commonly leads to Korsakoff's psychosis, a severe anterograde amnesia. (See *Effects of alcohol abuse,* page 120.)

Symptoms of *alcohol withdrawal* may include tremors, anxiety, diaphoresis, diarrhea, tachycardia, tachypnea, hyperpnea, vomiting, and fever. Onset occurs several hours after the patient's last drink. Symptoms usually peak in 24 to 48 hours. The patient may experience alcoholic seizures 7 to 48 hours after his last drink. Complications during withdrawal may cause death, especially if the patient suffers from pneumonia, liver failure, subdural hematomas, or other problems.

In alcohol withdrawal delirium (delirium tremens), the patient experiences confusion, disorientation, paranoid delusions, or visual or tactile hallucinations along with other symptoms of withdrawal.

Alcoholics also have an alarmingly high suicide rate, and alcohol use has been associated with such violent crimes as assault, rape, child molestation, and murder. Of course, intoxication causes numerous automobile-related injuries and deaths. In addition, individ-

Continued on page 120

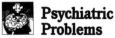
Substance Abuse and Eating Disorders

Alcoholism among women and the elderly

Alcoholism was once seen as a disease that primarily afflicted middle-aged men. Today, its influence cuts across the sexes and many age groups.

Women: Seeking psychological benefits

Statistics indicate that the number of female alcoholics will increase. Already, an estimated 10% of adult women in the U.S. show signs of alcohol dependency, and 5% have suffered adverse consequences related to drinking, such as conflicts with husbands, family, and friends; traffic accidents; or arrests for drunken driving.

Male and female alcoholics share similar personality traits and undergo similar stages in the course of illness. However, female alcoholics differ from their male counterparts in some important respects. For instance, they drink less frequently in public and are more likely to drink in response to stress. They also tend to develop alcoholism later in life.

Alcoholic women suffer from low self-esteem and feelings of powerlessness and incompetence, and frequently view drinking as a means to obtain psychological benefits. They frequently have a history of depression, sexual abuse or dysfunction, or divorce. More married working women develop alcoholism than single working women or housewives.

The elderly alcoholic: Alone and unnoticed

Alcoholism represents a far more common phenomenon among the elderly than most people realize. Increased tolerance to alcohol and excessive leisure time heighten the risk of problem drinking. Social drinking often escalates into alcoholism after retirement, especially for those with few outside interests or hobbies.

Because many elderly people live alone, alcoholism often goes unnoticed. Many take prescription drugs and remain uninformed about potentially dangerous interactions. Many visit several different doctors and obtain prescriptions for various mood-altering drugs. Be alert for symptoms of withdrawal when elderly patients enter the hospital.

Effects of alcohol abuse

Chronic alcohol abuse can lead to many physical and psychological complications, including the following:

Cardiovascular complications
- alcoholic cardiomyopathy
- increased systolic and pulse pressure
- tissue damage, weakened heart muscle, and heart failure

Gastrointestinal complications
- abdominal distention, pain, belching, and hematemesis
- acute and chronic pancreatitis
- alcoholic hepatitis leading to cirrhosis
- cancer of the esophagus, liver, or pancreas
- esophageal varices, hemorrhoids, and ascites
- gastritis, colitis, and enteritis
- stomach or duodenal ulcers
- swollen, enlarged fatty liver

Genitourinary complications
- swelling of prostate gland, leading to prostatitis and interference with voiding or sexual function
- prostate cancer

Hematologic complications
- abnormal red blood cells, white blood cells, and platelets
- anemia and increased risk of infection
- bleeding tendencies, increased bruising, and decreased clotting time

Neurologic complications
- Wernicke-Korsakoff syndrome, Marchiafava-Bignami disease, cerebellar degeneration, and peripheral neuropathy

Respiratory complications
- cancer of the oropharynx
- impaired diffusion, chronic obstructive pulmonary disease, infection, and tuberculosis
- respiratory depression causing decreased respiratory rate and cough reflex and increased susceptibility to infection and trauma

Miscellaneous complications
- acute and chronic myopathies
- alcoholic amblyopia
- beriberi
- electrolyte abnormalities
- osteoporosis
- scars, burns, and repeated injuries

Frequently abused substances—*continued*

uals frequently combine alcohol and drugs, resulting in deadly overdoses or undermedication. (See *Drug-alcohol interactions.*)

Assessment. Signs of alcohol abuse may include loss of inhibitions (a pseudostimulant effect that causes hyperactivity of primitive parts of the brain), disorganized thoughts, poor coordination, and unstable moods. Other signs include flushed face, slurred speech, prolonged reaction time, reduced visual acuity, blackouts, nystagmus, and disturbed sleep patterns (decreased REM sleep). Consider showing the patient a list of these signs and asking which he's experienced.

The following questions may help uncover more information on the patient's pattern of drinking:
- How often do you drink?
- What kinds of liquor do you drink? How much of each?
- How much alcohol do you consume each day?
- For how long have you consumed alcohol at this rate?
- How have your drinking habits changed over time?

Substance Abuse and Eating Disorders

Drug-alcohol interactions

Drug	Drug-alcohol effects
Analgesics Antianxiety drugs Antidepressants Antihistamines Antipsychotics Hypnotics	Deepened central nervous system (CNS) depression
Monoamine oxidase inhibitors	Deepened CNS depression. Possible hypertensive crisis with some beers and high-tyramine-content wines (Chianti, Alicante)
Sulfonylurea oral hypoglycemics	Disulfiram-like effects (facial flushing, headache), especially with chlorpropamide. If food intake isn't adequate, patient may experience increased hypoglycemic activity

Some antibacterial agents
  Cephalosporins
  Metronidazole
	Disulfiram-like effects

- When was your last drink?
- Has drinking created problems for you? If so, what are they?
- Have you ever experienced blackouts, tremors, delirium tremens, or seizures? When and for how long?
- Have you ever tried to stop drinking? If so, what happened?
- Have you experienced auditory, visual, or tactile hallucinations? Were you drinking heavily at the time? Describe the experience.
- Are you currently taking any prescription, over-the-counter, or illicit drugs? If so, what are they?
- Have you ever used illicit drugs?
- Are you married? Do you have children? Who lives with you? Has anyone close to you expressed concern over your alcohol use? Give details.
- Were you ever arrested for driving while intoxicated or for any other reason?
- Have you experienced problems at work or been unemployed for a significant amount of time?
- Have you ever enjoyed a sober period? When and for how long?
- Have you undergone treatment for alcoholism or medical or emotional problems before?
- Have you ever participated in Alcoholics Anonymous?

Information gathered during the interview may indicate what complications to expect during detoxification and treatment.

Diagnostic tests. More than 50% of alcoholics show increased levels of serum gamma-glutamyltransferase. Alcoholics also commonly show increased mean corpuscular volume, reduced white cell count, and elevated levels of uric acid, triglycerides, aspartate aminotransferase, and urea.

Assessing for alcoholic neuropathy. Alcoholic neuropathy usually appears between ages 40 and 70. Onset is slow, progressive, and insidious, involving multiple nerve degeneration. Ask the patient if he's experienced loss of reflexes or feeling or had tingling, prickling,

Continued on page 122

Substance Abuse and Eating Disorders

Assessing alcohol withdrawal

When assessing for alcohol withdrawal, use this checklist.
☐ History of long-term, heavy alcohol use
☐ History of withdrawal symptoms during previous cessation of drinking
☐ 8 or more hours since last drink
☐ Tremulousness, diaphoresis, anxiety, agitation
☐ Elevated pulse (110 beats/minute or greater) and blood pressure (150/90 mm Hg or higher)
☐ Possible fever
☐ Hallucinations
☐ Generalized tonic-clonic seizures without history of epilepsy

Possible associated conditions
☐ Nausea, vomiting, diarrhea
☐ Gastritis
☐ Liver injury
☐ Skin conditions (for example, psoriasis)
☐ Musculoskeletal injuries (secondary to trauma)
☐ Peripheral neuropathy
☐ Cognitive dysfunction
☐ Upper respiratory infection

Frequently abused substances—*continued*

burning, or numbness in his feet or hands. Ask about pain, pruritus, or loss of control or sensation in his legs and dull or sharp pains in his arm or leg joints. Assess for tenderness in the calves, weakness, a wide-stance gait, and diminished sensitivity to pain, temperature, or vibration.

Assessing for alcohol withdrawal. If you suspect a patient is about to undergo alcohol withdrawal, observe him closely. Monitor pulse and blood pressure every 2 hours for the first 12 hours, every 4 hours for the next 24 hours, and every 6 hours thereafter (more frequently if patient's unstable). Suspect alcohol withdrawal if the patient's pulse reaches or exceeds 110 beats/minute and his blood pressure is 150/90 mm Hg or higher without a coexisting illness.

Be alert for tremors, increased anxiety, and diaphoresis. Notify the doctor immediately of any signs of withdrawal. Early intervention can prevent dangerous reactions. (See *Assessing alcohol withdrawal.*)

Intervention. Help the patient through withdrawal. Whether or not he'll enter the hospital to go through withdrawal depends on the severity of symptoms, the stage of withdrawal, physical and emotional complications, the availability of alternative support services, and the patient's history and ability to comply with instructions.

Patients with mild withdrawal symptoms often do well in outpatient programs that feature daily follow-up visits and observation for complications. Patients who frequently require inpatient care include those with organic brain syndrome, low intelligence, Wernicke's encephalopathy, dehydration, previous head trauma, neurologic symptoms, complications, alcohol withdrawal delirium, seizures and hallucinations, or those taking psychotropic medications.

Detoxification works best in a structured unit with a supportive, nonjudgmental staff and a minimum of stimulation. Most inpatient programs use sedatives to make withdrawal more bearable and to prevent seizures and delerium tremens. Most likely, the doctor will order large, frequent doses of a cross-tolerant benzodiazepine to forestall severe withdrawal reactions. Relatively safe, benzodiazepines can be given orally or intravenously.

Usually, one benzodiazepine works as well as another, but chlordiazepoxide (Librium) is commonly the drug of choice. Elderly patients and those with severe liver disease, however, do better with an intermediate-acting benzodiazepine, such as lorazepam (Ativan) or oxazepam (Serax), that's excreted by the kidneys instead of by the liver. Patients addicted to other depressants and those who have a history of seizures do better on diazepam because of its anticonvulsant effects.

As the patient's vital signs stabilize, the doctor will decrease the sedative dosage gradually over 3 to 5 days. Then he'll discontinue the drug.

During withdrawal, maintaining a calm environment may help prevent delerium tremens or ease the patient who has them. To maintain a calm environment:
• Keep intrusions to a minimimum.
• Move slowly and deliberately.

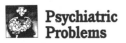
Substance Abuse and Eating Disorders

- Speak slowly and calmly, and call the patient by his name.
- Keep lighting even to prevent shadows and soft enough to prevent glare.
- Encourage a friend or family member to sit quietly with the patient and instruct them to call you should a problem arise.

Continue to check vital signs and behavior. Try to keep the patient oriented. If he hallucinates, reorient him to reality. During and after withdrawal, the patient will require oral thiamine, folic acid, and multivitamins to correct nutritional deficiencies, along with adequate food and fluids.

Disulfiram therapy. Used only infrequently, this therapy serves mainly as an adjunct to treatment in inpatient settings. Disulfiram inhibits the final pathways in alcohol metabolism. This causes buildup of acetaldehyde, resulting in moderate to severe systemic reactions to alcohol. Of course, patients taking disulfiram should be warned to avoid all foods and substances containing alcohol.

Opioids

Opioids include drugs derived from the poppy plant, such as heroin and morphine, as well as synthetic drugs, such as meperidine (Demerol), codeine, and methadone. These drugs induce analgesia, euphoria, or a dreamy drowsiness.

Teenagers and young adults constitute the most frequent abusers of heroin, the most popular opioid. They may band together into a subculture, encouraging each other's drug dependency and sharing techniques for enjoying the drug rush. To support expensive habits, they turn to dealing, theft, prostitution, or other illegal means. Dealers often add impurities to heroin (called cutting the drug), leading to poisoning and unexpected reactions. In addition, I.V. drug users who share needles face a high risk of contracting acquired immunodeficiency syndrome (AIDS) and hepatitis.

Other risks of opioid abuse include respiratory arrest, overdose, pulmonary edema, malnutrition, and death. Users commonly become physically addicted, and withdrawal symptoms usually appear within 12 hours after the last dose. The most severe symptoms occur within 48 hours, decreasing gradually over the next 2 weeks. During withdrawal, the patient experiences intense craving for the drug.

Assessment. Look for signs of abuse, such as impaired attention span and memory, euphoria, sedation ("nodding out"), psychomotor retardation, insensitivity to pain, agitation, apathy, or dysphoria. Also look for pinpoint pupils (except with meperidine), slurred speech, nausea and vomiting, and hypothermia. If the patient abuses I.V. drugs, you may notice local abscesses or signs of subacute bacterial endocarditis caused by sloppy injection technique or sharing of needles.

Behavioral clues to opiate addiction may include disinterest in hygiene and appearance, preoccupation with drugs, a criminal record, poor judgment, frequent accidents, drunken gait and behavior, and impulsiveness.

Be alert for withdrawal symptoms. These may include dilated pupils, tearing eyes, runny nose, piloerection, sweating, diarrhea, fever,

Continued on page 125

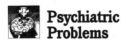
Substance Abuse and Eating Disorders

Commonly abused substances

Besides cocaine and heroin, other prescription and nonprescription drugs are commonly abused.

Barbiturates

Commonly prescribed barbiturates include phenobarbital (Luminal) and secobarbital (Seconal). These drugs vary in onset and duration of effects, depending on the amount taken and whether other drugs are taken concurrently.

Tolerance develops quickly, so the user constantly needs more of the drug to achieve the desired effect. Withdrawal produces severe symptoms. In fact, abrupt withdrawal can cause life-threatening seizures and delirium tremens (DTs). Long-term use can cause severe anxiety, tension, irritability, and problems with concentration and coordination. Permanent liver and pancreas damage may occur. Other problems include the risk of poisoning or overdose from street drugs laced with other substances and congenital birth defects from use during pregnancy.

Nonbarbiturate sedatives

Tranquilizers such as diazepam (Valium) and chlordiazepoxide (Librium) constitute the most commonly abused prescription drugs. Used to control anxiety, they may cause complicated or paradoxic adverse effects and may jeopardize long-term well-being. Withdrawal may cause general discomfort, profuse perspiration, vomiting, seizures, or DTs, and is potentially fatal.

The most common nonbarbiturate sedative used illegally today, methaqualone produces a pleasant effect, but it has a high potential for psychological and physical dependence. Once one of the most widely prescribed antianxiety drugs in the United States, it's no longer available by prescription. Concurrent use with alcohol or other sedatives may cause overdose or death.

Because methaqualone is manufactured illegally, the drug's potency and purity remain unknown. It may contain additional drugs such as diazepam, phenobarbital, antihistamines, diphenhydramine (Benadryl), doxylamine (Unisom), acetaminophen (Tylenol), salicylamide (Uromide), ketamine (Ketalar), decongestants, phencyclidine, or look-alike substances, such as lactose (milk sugar). Before 1983, methaqualone was manufactured under the trade name Quaalude.

Amphetamines

The most common of these central nervous system stimulants are methamphetamine (Desoxyn) and dextroamphetamine (Dexedrine). Their use as prescription diet aids has declined, but illegal use has increased. Truck drivers, students studying for exams, factory workers, and people seeking stimulation or extra energy may rely on them. Abuse may lead to numerous adverse effects, including acute amphetamine psychosis (5% to 15% of patients don't recover completely), aggressiveness, dysrhythmias, chills, seizures, decreased appetite, delirium, delusions, depression, and hypervigilance.

Marijuana

Made from the hemp plant *Cannabis sativa,* marijuana creates a high that lasts for 2 or 3 hours. Its active ingredient is delta-9-tetrahydrocannabinol (THC). THC can be detected in fatty tissue up to 6 weeks after use. The drug's effect depends on its strength as well as the individual's psychological state and surrounding environment. Possible mood-altering drug effects include distortion of time, reality, or perception and impairment of short-term memory.

Recent studies do not completely bear out the popular notion that marijuana use is innocuous. Long-term use in men can lower sperm count and increase the number of abnormally shaped sperm. The drug might also affect the female reproductive system. Inhaling marijuana smoke can also cause lung disease.

Hallucinogenics

Synthetic and natural hallucinogenic drugs provide unusual sensory experiences. During the 1960s, LSD use became popular as a means of achieving insight and sensory awareness. However, the drug lost popularity after several well-publicized accidental deaths related to its use. Today, teenagers use the drug to obtain an inexpensive, intense high that lasts up to 12 hours. Other hallucinogenics include psilocybin, PCP, DMT, mescaline, peyote, and MDA.

Hallucinogenics create a crossover from one sensory modality to another, creating the sensation of "hearing" color and "seeing" sound. Risks include the potential for a "bad trip" accompanied by intense feelings of fear, anxiety, and paranoia as well as the danger of chromosomal changes.

Phencyclidine (PCP). In small doses, PCP raises blood pressure and heart rate and may cause agitation, hallucinations, violence, psychosis, and even coma and death. Developed as an animal anesthetic, the drug may be legally obtained only by veterinarians. Home chemists manufacture it for street use.

You may encounter patients overdosing on PCP when working in the emergency department. The doctor may order diazepam or haloperidol (Haldol) to control severe psychotic behavior; however, because PCP is anticholinergic, phenothiazines such as thorazine aren't used. Psychologists believe that schizophrenics are especially sensitive to the drug's effects.

Inhalants

Individuals may achieve a high by sniffing or inhaling solvents and aerosols, such as gasoline fumes, glue, lacquer-thinner, lighter fluid, deodorants, hair spray, and paint. Amyl nitrite (for treatment of angina) and butyl nitrite (sold over the counter) may be inhaled from cloth or plastic bags or directly from their containers.

Fat-soluble chemicals that depress respiration and pulse rates, inhalants produce an initial sense of well-being. Potential adverse effects include nosebleeds, bloodshot eyes, bad breath, sores on the mouth and nose, unconsciousness, and seizures. Potentially fatal reactions include myocardial infarction caused by irregular heartbeat, suffocation caused by passing out when breathing into a plastic bag, and depressed bone marrow function leading to aplastic anemia.

Substance Abuse and Eating Disorders

Street names for abused drugs

Barbiturates
Thrill pills, downers, goof balls, reds, red birds, red devils, yellow jackets, blue heavens, rainbows

Methaqualone
Ludes, 714s, quall, love drug, mandrake, lemons, sopers, quads

Heroin
Horse, smack, junk, scag, stuff

Amphetamines
Speed, dynamite, lidpoppers, white crosses, hearts, co-pilots, bennies, jolly beans, dexies, crystal, meth

Marijuana
Pot, grass, weed, Mary Jane, roach, reefer, joint

Cocaine
Coke, blow, cosmos, crack, colombo, flake, and snow. *Look-alike substances are called* Florida snow, cocaine snuff, coco snow, milky trail, rock crystal, and ultra caine

PCP
Angel dust, crystal superjoint, hog, elephant tranquilizer, THC, rocket fuel, peace pill

Inhalants
Poppers, snappers, pearls, amys, popsies, jacaroma, jac-blaster, locker room, black-jac, rush, bullet, crypt, aroma of man

Frequently abused substances—*continued*

yawning, mild hypotension, tachycardia, insomnia, restlessness and irritability, muscle and joint pain, increased respiration, GI symptoms, and loss of appetite.

Interventions. Many heroin addicts turn to methadone maintenance programs to help them lead more productive lives and to ease the withdrawal process. Methadone alleviates the craving for narcotics and costs less than heroin, thereby helping them to avoid illegal activity. Expect to administer methadone in a liquid form in juice and to gradually decrease the dosage and eventually withdraw the drug.

Researchers are investigating the use of clonidine hydrochloride (Catapres), a nonopiate hypotensive drug that may hasten withdrawal and render it less painful. The patient receives methadone for 3 to 5 days and usually experiences withdrawal within 1 to 3 days after discontinuing methadone. The doctor then administers clonidine until withdrawal symptoms dissipate.

Nursing measures for a patient undergoing withdrawal include maintaining hydration, either by infusing fluids or by offering frequent fluids that don't worsen GI irritation or impair motility. Other interventions include keeping the patient warm and maintaining a calm, nonstimulating environment. If the patient suffers from prolonged, severe diarrhea, administer antidiarrhea medication as ordered.

To help postwithdrawal patients stay opioid free, the doctor may order naltrexone. This opiate antagonist deprives the former addict of a high should he go back to using opioids. Warn the patient not to try to overcome naltrexone's effects by taking large doses of narcotics, because they may cause serious injury, coma, or death. Explain that naltrexone doesn't produce tolerance or dependency.

Overdose. Symptoms of opioid-induced overdose include fixed pupillary constrictions, respiratory depression (less than 6 respirations per minute), and coma. If a patient overdoses, administer 0.4 to 0.8 mg I.V. of naloxone (Narcan), repeated in 5 to 15 minutes. A fast-acting narcotic antagonist, naloxone counteracts respiratory depression. Belladonna alkaloids or phenobarbital may treat abdominal cramps, rhinorrhea, and lacrimation.

Cocaine

A stimulant derived from the coca plant, cocaine achieved phenomenal popularity in the 1980s, beginning as a chic expensive drug for young upwardly mobile professionals before filtering down to all cultural and socioeconomic groups. Users now span the range from inner-city teenagers to top executives, equally divided between men and women.

The cocaine user experiences an intense euphoria, followed by a strong craving to repeat the high. He may also report such benefits as accelerated thinking, intensified awareness, increased self-confidence, and improved sexual performance. For about 2 weeks after his last dose, the cocaine user may suffer from abstinence syndrome ("postcoke blues")—terrible feelings of anxiety, depression, fatigue,

Continued on page 126

Substance Abuse and Eating Disorders

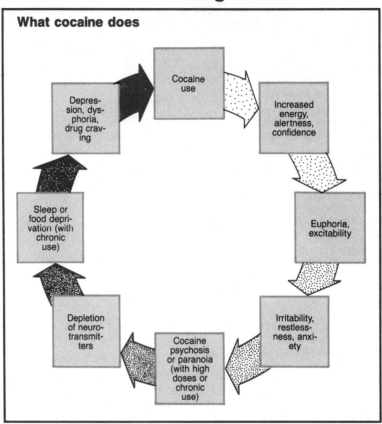

What cocaine does

Cocaine use → Increased energy, alertness, confidence → Euphoria, excitability → Irritability, restlessness, anxiety → Cocaine psychosis or paranoia (with high doses or chronic use) → Depletion of neurotransmitters → Sleep or food deprivation (with chronic use) → Depression, dysphoria, drug craving → Cocaine use

Frequently abused substances—*continued*

and insomnia that reinforce the craving for the drug. With frequent use, the cocaine high becomes more and more difficult to obtain. (See *What cocaine does*.)

Users may snort, smoke, chew, inject, or freebase cocaine. Freebasing refers to a chemical process using ether that allows the user to inhale a pure form of cocaine. It carries an added risk of singeing the eyebrows or eyelashes or even causing explosion. I.V. cocaine users who share needles risk contracting AIDS or hepatitis. Because dealers often adulterate cocaine with synthetic methamphetamine or other look-alike substances that produce mind-altering effects, users may suffer hallucinations and temporary psychosis. Cocaine also depletes stores of the neurotransmitters dopamine and norepinephrine. Complications include syncope, fever, chest pain, and potentially fatal seizures, dysrhythmias, or respiratory arrest.

In recent years, a new highly potent form of cocaine called *crack* has become widely used. Crack consists of cocaine hydrochloride mixed with baking soda. After hardening, the mixture is broken into small pieces and smoked in cigarettes or glass water pipes. More insidious and toxic than cocaine, crack is inexpensive and readily available. It rapidly produces intense euphoria followed by a dramatic crash. Seconds later, the user feels compelled to smoke more crack. Addiction occurs rapidly, and treatment centers now have long waiting lists. Experts estimate recidivism at 90%. Symptoms of crack use include irritability, paranoia, and depression. Wheezing and coughing blood and black phlegm may result from smoking toxins. Dysrhythmias caused by crack may lead to death.

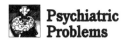
Substance Abuse and Eating Disorders

Assessment. Look for signs of cocaine abuse, such as psychomotor agitation, anxiety, assaultive behavior, increased alertness and activity, talkativeness, grandiosity, hypervigilance, impaired judgment, ideas of reference, paranoid hallucinations, formication (sensation of insects crawling on the skin), euphoria followed by depression, insomnia, or anorexia. The patient may also need sedatives to sleep, especially if he uses other illicit drugs.

Other signs of abuse may include dilated pupils, tachycardia, elevated blood pressure, perspiration, hyperpyrexia, chills, nausea, vomiting, anorexia, dry mouth, bad breath, weight loss, stuffy or runny nose, tremors, muscle cramping, and seizures. Long-term use may lead to damaged nasal mucosa, tolerance, malnutrition, and cardiac irregularities.

Intervention. Still in the experimental phase, detoxification for cocaine abusers depends upon hospital protocol and the patient's symptoms. I.V. diazepam may help control seizures, decrease vomiting, and reduce stimulation. Treatment may last for about 4 days, with the dosage gradually decreased. The doctor may order additional doses if the patient experiences withdrawal symptoms. I.V. ammonium chloride may enhance cocaine excretion.

Other detoxification regimens consist of phenobarbital in decreasing doses and imipramine hydrochloride (Tofranil). Note, however, that not all hospitals will medicate cocaine abusers.

To control severe depression, the doctor may order tricyclic antidepressants, such as imipramine or amitriptyline (Elavil), for several weeks after detoxification. These drugs work by enhancing the effects of the remaining neurotransmitters.

Amino acids such as tyrosine, phenylalanine, cysteine, or glutamic acid may help to alleviate depression and fatigue during withdrawal. These amino acids are converted to neurotransmitters, replenishing the body's depleted supply. Tryptophan may also curb depression and drug craving and promote sleep.

To combat psychotic symptoms, the doctor may order haloperidol (Haldol). Phenothiazines, which may decrease the patient's seizure threshold, should be avoided.

Keep in mind that even small doses of cocaine may cause life-threatening effects. Focus treatment on preventing progression of symptoms. For example, if the patient shows signs of hyperpyrexia, begin cooling procedures to prevent seizures.

To treat cocaine-induced dysrhythmia, the doctor may order propranolol, lidocaine, or calcium channel blockers. Nifedipine has also been found effective in combatting cocaine's cardiotoxic effects.

Eating disorders

Individuals may turn to other substances besides drugs and alcohol to help with life's problems. In fact, food may represent the most commonly abused substance. Its unhealthful use can lead to three potentially life-threatening disorders: Anorexia nervosa, bulimia nervosa, and obesity. (See *Obesity,* page 128.)

Continued on page 128

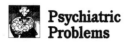

Substance Abuse and Eating Disorders

Eating disorders—*continued*

Anorexia nervosa

An eating disorder characterized by self-imposed starvation, anorexia nervosa affects 1 in 250 women between the ages of 12 and 18. Men account for about 5% of anorectic patients. Characteristically, the patient shows signs of extreme weight loss to the point of emaciation. Women commonly experience amenorrhea, often before weight loss becomes noticeable. (See *Anorexia nervosa: Physical signs*.)

Psychologists have suggested various causes of anorexia nervosa, such as fear of growing up and sexually maturing. In such patients, anorexia may offer a way to express conflicts over sexual identity. Another possible cause may reflect sociocultural values. In the past few decades, society's ideal feminine shape has become increasingly lean and angular; consequently, women have become increasingly preoccupied with losing weight.

Some psychologists attribute the disorder to emotional distress brought on by a controlling, domineering mother and an absent or emotionally distant father. Others have cited organic problems, including electrolyte imbalances or enlarged ventricles in the brain.

Assessment. Focus on the patient's attitude toward food, her lifestyle, and her eating habits. Expect her to express an intense fear of gaining weight and to deny the obvious signs of her condition.

Look for indications of peculiar eating habits. The patient may collect recipes and prepare elaborate meals for family members. At meals, she may cut her food into small pieces, then rearrange the scraps

Obesity

Just as an alcoholic loses control over drinking, an obese patient loses control over eating. Energy (caloric) intake exceeds energy expenditure, causing storage of excess energy in the form of fat.

What causes obesity?

In addition to overeating, several other factors may influence obesity. Complicated neural mechanisms that control appetite and various metabolic processes affect eating behavior. Obese people frequently complain that they can't stop eating or never feel satiated. Some also confuse other dysphoric states with hunger.

Heredity also seems to influence obesity. About 80% of children with two obese parents are themselves obese, compared to 40% of children with one obese parent and only 10% of children with parents of normal weight. Studies of twins and adoptees support this theory.

Obese people also have larger fat cells and more of them. Fat cells usually multiply early in life, but they can grow in size in adulthood. The process that controls fat-cell growth remains unknown.

Lack of exercise also contributes to obesity. Although relatively few calories are expended through exercise, animal studies show that exercise decreases appetite and may also prevent the decrease in metabolic rate that accompanies dieting.

Intervention

The most effective treatment for *mild obesity* (20% to 40% above normal weight) is behavior modification, support groups, a balanced diet, and exercise.

Moderate obesity (41% to 100% above normal weight) may require a medically supervised, protein-sparing, modified fast with 400 to 700 calories a day. Before the patient begins a behavior modification program, he may undergo an analysis of his eating behavior. Treatment programs may combine self-monitoring, nutrition education, physical activity, and cognitive restructuring. Medications such as phenylpropanolamine (Acutrim) and fenfluramine (Pondimin) may also help moderately obese patients lose weight. However, many patients regain weight and feel lethargic and depressed upon discontinuing these drugs.

Patients with *severe obesity* (more than 100% over normal weight) may benefit from surgical procedures that reduce the size of the stomach. Patients usually maintain the large weight loss that results.

Psychotherapy

Many obese people become depressed when they attempt to diet. Many also suffer from the social stigma attached to being overweight. But studies have not shown depression to be any more prevalent in obese people than in the general population. And while psychotherapy may help some obese patients with emotional problems, it does not constitute by itself a treatment for obesity.

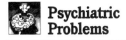
Substance Abuse and Eating Disorders

Look for the following characteristic signs when assessing anorectic patients:
• Extreme weight loss and emaciated, unhealthy appearance
• Loss of secondary sex characteristics (for example, loss of pubic hair, shrinking of breasts)
• Cessation of menses
• Muscle weakness
• Early morning awakening
• Anemia
• Coldness
• Cyanosis
• Dry hands and feet
• Lanugo
• Constipation
• Electrolyte imbalance
• Bradycardia, dysrhythmias, hypotension, cardiac arrest

on her plate or surreptitiously dispose of them. Her obsession with food may remind you of an addict's preoccupation with drugs. When eating, however, she'll limit herself to small quantities of low-calorie foods, such as lettuce.

Other common characteristics in anorectics include:
• obsessive-compulsive behavior; frequently a high achiever, the patient may become preoccupied with cleaning, studying, or other activity
• habitual mirror gazing
• concern with self-control; the patient may equate controlling weight with achieving self-discipline
• repeated statements, such as "I'm getting fat," that reveal her distorted self-image
• vigorous exercise, to gain even more control over body weight
• purging through self-induced vomiting, laxatives, or diuretics
• poor sexual adjustment; adolescents may have delayed sexual development, and adults may have little interest in sex.

Intervention. Often the anorectic patient seeks treatment only after her condition becomes life threatening. If so, focus on renourishing the patient. In extreme cases, the patient may require total parenteral nutrition.

Once the patient begins eating on her own, behavior modification may help reinforce healthful nutrition. Rewards for eating substantially may include television or visitor privileges. Of course, make sure the patient understands your expectations, or else such treatment may appear unfair or punitive.

The patient may be indifferent or resistant to treatment. If her condition begins to improve, she may complain about getting fat or losing control over eating habits. Reassure the patient that you won't let her overeat and become obese. As treatment progresses, focus attention on the underlying psychological conflicts. The patient may benefit from individual, group, or family therapy.

Bulimia nervosa

Also known as anorexia bulimia or simply as bulimia, this disorder is characterized by binge eating followed by self-induced vomiting. During a binge, patients consume large quantities of such high-calorie foods as ice cream, cake, doughnuts, and bread—perhaps as much as 5,000 calories at a sitting. Binge eating usually lasts for about an hour; then abdominal pain, self-induced vomiting, sleep, or an interruption stops it. At first, patients vomit by sticking their fingers down their throats, but eventually they vomit reflexively. They may also use laxatives or diuretics to prevent weight gain. The disorder is thought to have reached near-epidemic proportions among young women.

Researchers have described bulimia as a primary neurologic disturbance similar to epilepsy, as a hypothalamic disturbance, as a conditioned response to stress, and as an inability to suppress an oral urge.

Assessment. Bulimic patients usually don't exhibit obvious signs. Unlike anorectics, many appear to be of normal weight. Furthermore, patients binge and purge in secret.

Continued on page 130

Substance Abuse and Eating Disorders

Eating disorders—*continued*

Attempt to gain insight into the patient's eating patterns. Keep in mind that, besides binging and purging, most bulimic patients diet, either successfully or unsuccessfully, for a few weeks or several months before the disorder's onset. Typically, they don't eat regular meals or feel satisfied after a normal meal. They prefer eating at home, alone.

Check for signs of anxiety and depression. After a binge, bulimics feel guilty, depressed, and disgusted with themselves. Many report feeling helpless to stop a binge. Many also report problems forming interpersonal relationships.

Check for a history of chemical dependency; bulimics frequently abuse alcohol or take amphetamines to curb their appetite. Also check for a history of compulsive stealing. Typically, stealing occurs after a binge episode, with patients taking food, clothing, and jewelry.

Assess for signs of induced vomiting, such as erosion of dental enamel and finger abrasions on the dominant hand. Check for other signs of bulimia, such as esophagitis, dilated abdomen, and hypokalemia.

Intervention. Focus on helping the patient control binge eating and other inappropriate impulses. Unfortunately, research has yet to uncover effective treatment, although antidepressants, anticonvulsants, and psychotherapy (especially group therapy) may help.

Consider the individual patient's condition. Many bulimics also have diagnoses of borderline personality disorder, drug or alcohol dependence, post-traumatic stress syndrome, or depression. Give priority to any serious medical problems or indications of suicide.

Before a binge episode, patients report various anxiety-related feelings, including anger and frustration at their inability to meet other's expectations. Help them explore and gain control of these feelings and thereby achieve greater confidence and self-control. Effective management of prodromal feelings will help curb the onset of future binge episodes.

Personality Disorders: Antisocial and Borderline

Kem B. Louie, a psychotherapist in private practice in Rutherford, N.J., wrote this chapter. Also an assistant professor at the Lehman College of City University of New York, Bronx, N.Y., she received her BSN from Rutgers College of Nursing, Newark, N.J., and her MA and PhD from New York University.

Personality disorder refers to a chronic pattern of inflexible, maladaptive traits that influence a patient's affect, cognition, behavior, and style of interacting with others. It causes severe personal distress and impairs social and occupational function.

Typically, the patient with a personality disorder has had difficulty with emotional development during early childhood. Symptoms often appear by childhood or adolescence and make it difficult to cope with the demands of everyday life. The disorder may result from ineffective or absent parents, early childhood experiences, temperament at birth, or genetic and biochemical factors. Although factors like these influence everyone's personality development, the patient with a personality disorder develops an unhealthful pattern of interaction that becomes fixed.

Dealing with an affected patient requires not only sensitivity to his feelings, but also insight into your own emotions. Such a patient commonly provokes strong reactions. For instance, you may become filled with empathy and kindness for him when he expresses feelings of helplessness and isolation. Your warm feelings, however, may quickly give way to frustration when the patient refuses to take the smallest steps to help himself. Preventing your frustration from interfering with proper care requires careful self-assessment.

The revised third edition of the *Diagnostic and Statistical Manual of Mental Disorders* (DSM-III-R) groups personality disorders into three types, based on their dominant traits. (See *Classifying personality disorders*, page 132.) Recently, the DSM-III-R has listed two other personality disorders: sadistic and self-defeating personality disorders. (See *Opposite personality problems*, page 133.)

This chapter focuses on antisocial and borderline personality disorders. In a general hospital setting, patients with these disorders are likely to provoke especially strong feelings from members of the health care team, and their behavior often disrupts care.

Antisocial personality disorder

Sometimes termed sociopathic or psychopathic behavior, antisocial personality disorder affects an estimated 3% of men and less than 1% of women in the United States. It occurs most commonly among lower socioeconomic groups. This may be partly explained by the fact that patients commonly can't hold a job.

The patient with antisocial personality disorder lacks empathy, fails to form significant attachments, and displays concern only for his own needs. He persistently violates others' rights, demonstrates no guilt or remorse, and disregards the consequences of his behavior. Typically, he doesn't voluntarily seek psychological treatment and may enter the hospital as an emergency room or surgical patient or to seek treatment for substance abuse.

Causes: Several theories
According to some psychologists, antisocial personality disorder often goes unrecognized because of the patient's convincing "mask of sanity." The disorder does not produce the outward signs com-

Continued on page 133

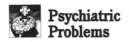
Personality Disorders

Classifying personality disorders

TYPE AND DISORDER		CHARACTERISTICS
TYPE A: ODD, ECCENTRIC	**Paranoid**	• Pervasive, unwarranted mistrust of others, manifested by jealousy, envy, and guardedness • Hypersensitivity, frequent feelings of being mistreated and misjudged • Restricted affect, evidenced by lack of tenderness and poor sense of humor
	Schizoid	• Inability to form social relationships, absence of warm and tender feeling for others • Indifference to praise, criticism, and feelings of others • Apparently little or no desire for social involvement; usually few, if any, close friends • Generally reserved, withdrawn, and seclusive; preference for solitary interests or hobbies • Dull or flat affect, appears cold or aloof
	Schizotypal	• Various oddities of thought, perception, speech, and behavior not severe enough to warrant a diagnosis of schizophrenia • Possible magical thinking, ideas of reference, paranoid ideation, illusions, depersonalization, peculiarities in word choice, social isolation, and inappropriate affect
TYPE B: DRAMATIC, EMOTIONAL, ERRATIC, IMPULSIVE	**Antisocial**	• General disregard for others' rights and feelings • History of persistent antisocial behavior, such as lying, fighting, stealing, vandalism, truancy, impulsive and reckless behavior, substance abuse, and promiscuity • Poor school or job performance record • Inability to maintain close interpersonal relationships, especially a sexually intimate one • Superficial charm, often with manipulative and seductive behavior
	Borderline	• Instability in interpersonal behavior, marked by intense and unstable relationships • Impulsive and unpredictable behavior • Profound, inappropriate shifts in mood and affect • Poor identity with uncertainty in such areas as self-image, sexual preference, values, and future goals
	Histrionic	• Lively, dramatic, attention-seeking behavior • Tantrums and angry outbursts • Demanding, egocentric, inconsiderate behavior • Manipulation and divisiveness • Seductive or charming behavior • Superficial personal attachments
	Narcissistic	• Exaggerated sense of self-importance, manifested by extreme self-centeredness • Preoccupation with fantasies involving power, success, wealth, beauty, or love • No capacity for empathy • Need for constant admiration and attention • Manipulative behavior
TYPE C: ANXIOUS, FEARFUL	**Avoidant**	• Anxiety and fearfulness • Low self-esteem • Hypersensitivity to potential humiliation, rejection, or shame • Social withdrawal accompanied by longing for close relationships
	Dependent	• Extreme self-consciousness, accompanied by feelings of inadequacy and helplessness • Dependency in relationships, subordinating own needs and leaving major decisions to others • Overly passive and compliant
	Compulsive	• Inability to express affection • Overly cold and rigid demeanor • Preoccupation with rules, trivial details, and other expressions of conformity • Superior attitude • Need to control • Tendency toward perfection, valuing work more than pleasure or relationships
	Passive-aggressive	• Intentional inefficiency in social and occupational function, marked by chronic lateness, procrastination, and forgetfulness • Resentment, sullenness, and stubbornness unaccompanied by overt hostility • Fear of authority

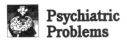
Personality Disorders

Opposite personality problems

Compared to each other, sadistic and self-defeating personality disorders represent the opposite ends of the spectrum of personality problems.

Sadistic personality disorder
The patient with sadistic personality disorder may humiliate others in private or in public, enforce overly harsh discipline on individuals under his control, take pleasure in the psychological or physical suffering of others (including animals), or commit acts of violence, aggression, exploitation, or even terror. He doesn't use violence to achieve some impersonal goal, but views cruelty and domination as an end in itself.

The patient is likely to dominate friends and family and may restrict their movements, for example, by refusing to allow them to attend social functions outside the home. He may collect weapons, martial arts paraphernalia, and books or videotapes with violent themes. This behavior is directed toward more than one individual and is not solely for the purpose of sexual arousal.

Self-defeating personality disorder
In this disorder, the affected patient is resigned to failure, suffering, and exploitation. He believes his misfortunes are justified and willingly places himself in harmful relationships.

When people reach out to the patient, he rejects or ignores their efforts. Following success, he experiences depression and guilt and reverts to self-defeating behavior. Despite demonstrated ability, he often fails to accomplish his objectives. He may deliberately provoke anger from an acquaintance and later feel rejected and hurt. He's loathe to acknowledge the few occasions when he does enjoy himself. He acts submissive and self-sacrificing, regardless of whether others want or expect such acquiescence. These behaviors don't occur only during periods of depression.

Antisocial personality disorder—*continued*

monly associated with psychiatric problems, such as loss of cognitive processes, unusual verbal or facial expressions, or lability of affect. What sets the patient apart is his inability to feel common human emotions. Because of this inability, he has only a superficial understanding of others' feelings and motivations. (See *Stages of moral development,* page 134.)

In contrast, other psychologists contend that the patient, far from having no feelings, is actually overwhelmed by his emotions and struggles to keep them out of his consciousness. He may develop a deep-rooted fear of close interpersonal relationships after experiencing physical or emotional abuse or neglect during childhood. His apparent lack of emotion represents an elaborate defense against terrifying feelings, and his antisocial behavior represents a defense against the painful but persistent yearning for lost parental love.

Genetic factors may play a role in development of antisocial personality disorder as well. Studies indicate that a child whose biological father has antisocial personality disorder faces an increased risk, even if adopted when very young. Other studies suggest a link between serotonin and norepinephrine levels and the aggressive behavior that often characterizes antisocial persons. Serotonin is thought to decrease aggressive drives; norepinephrine, to sustain them. An antisocial person may have an imbalance of these substances as a result of genetic or environmental factors, or both.

Another theory suggests that antisocial personality disorder is an outgrowth of childhood attention deficit disorder, which may be an organic disturbance. In addition, the antisocial patient may have a defect in the autonomic nervous system that prevented him from feeling fear during childhood. As a result, he learned not to fear punishment and, therefore, has come to lack the motivation for modifying his behavior to socially acceptable standards.

Assessment
Identifying the disorder requires evidence of a persistent pattern of antisocial behavior. Psychological evaluation must rule out similar personality or other psychiatric disorders.

During your interview with the patient, take note of his behavior. Is he irritable, aggressive, threatening, or verbally abusive? Does he make a point to violate hospital rules? Note if he attempts to control the interview by intimidation, flattery, or deceit. To get his way, the patient may manipulate others, turn on a seductive charm, or make outright demands. Also note if he purposefully isolates himself or rejects friendly overtures.

You may also notice signs of personal distress, including complaints of anxiety or tension or inability to tolerate boredom or depression. The patient may talk of loneliness or feel, often not without justification, that others are hostile toward him.

Explore the patient's upbringing. Many patients have separated, divorced, ungiving, or abusive parents or parents who burdened their children with unrealistic expectations. Many also come from chaotic households or grew up in institutions or foster homes.

Continued on page 134

Personality Disorders

Antisocial personality disorder may indicate a breakdown during childhood in any of six stages of moral development shown here.

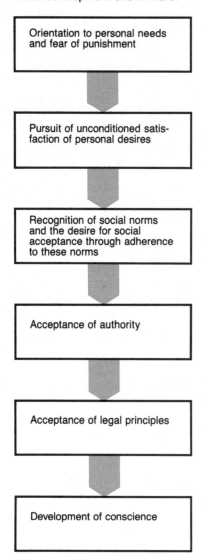

```
┌─────────────────────────────┐
│ Orientation to personal needs│
│ and fear of punishment       │
└─────────────────────────────┘
              ▼
┌─────────────────────────────┐
│ Pursuit of unconditioned     │
│ satisfaction of personal     │
│ desires                      │
└─────────────────────────────┘
              ▼
┌─────────────────────────────┐
│ Recognition of social norms  │
│ and the desire for social    │
│ acceptance through adherence │
│ to these norms               │
└─────────────────────────────┘
              ▼
┌─────────────────────────────┐
│ Acceptance of authority      │
└─────────────────────────────┘
              ▼
┌─────────────────────────────┐
│ Acceptance of legal principles│
└─────────────────────────────┘
              ▼
┌─────────────────────────────┐
│ Development of conscience     │
└─────────────────────────────┘
```

This breakdown explains the gap between the patient's knowledge and behavior. Although he can state the difference between right and wrong, he disregards the distinction.

Antisocial personality disorder—*continued*

Explore the patient's childhood for such problems as stealing, persistent lying, fighting, vandalism, truancy, running away from home, arson, or physical cruelty to animals or other children. Investigate behavior during adolescence, focusing on tobacco use, drug or alcohol abuse, and early sexual activity. Check for a history of somatization disorder.

In the adult patient, look for indications of impaired social and occupational function. The patient may have a poor job performance record or a noticeable lack of meaningful interpersonal relationships. He may fail to honor financial obligations, neglect to plan for the future, or disregard his responsibilities as a parent. Try to verify if he has a criminal record or uses illegal means to obtain a livelihood. Note any indications that he has engaged in destruction of property, harassment, stealing, assault, spouse- or child-beating, or drunken or reckless driving.

Ask the patient if he's concerned about his personal safety. Also ask if he feels remorseful about the effects of his behavior on others, and whether he feels justified in having hurt or mistreated friends or family.

After age 30, more flagrant antisocial acts, such as sexual promiscuity, fighting, and criminality, may diminish. However, interpersonal difficulties and dysphoria often continue into late adulthood. Almost invariably, the patient remains unable to sustain lasting relationships with family, friends, or sexual partners.

Diagnostic tests. Psychologists use three major tests to diagnose and evaluate personality disorders: the Minnesota Multiphasic Personality Inventory (MMPI), the Millon clinical multiaxial inventory, and the personality diagnostic questionnaire. Other tests are available to measure symptoms of specific personality disorders.

The MMPI may not provide the best method to identify and differentiate among the personality disorders listed in DSM-III-R. Research on the MMPI's usefulness in evaluating antisocial, borderline, and schizotypal personality disorders has yielded mixed results. Researchers have developed a new set of MMPI scales to evaluate personality disorders, but their effectiveness has yet to be confirmed.

The Millon clinical multiaxial inventory—much shorter and easier to administer than the MMPI—was developed in accordance with Millon's personality disorder taxonomy, which coincides with the DSM-III-R personality disorder classifications.

The personality diagnostic questionnaire, developed specifically to measure the personality disorders listed in DSM-III-R, contains much less overlap among the scales than does either the MMPI or the Millon clinical multiaxial inventory.

Planning

When planning your care, focus on reinforcing the patient's awareness of reality and discouraging him from manipulating others. Before determining your nursing care plan, develop the nursing diagnosis by identifying the patient's problem or potential problem, then relating it to its cause. Possible nursing diagnoses for a patient with antisocial personality disorder include:

Personality Disorders

Sample nursing care plan: Antisocial personality disorder

Nursing diagnosis	Expected outcomes
• Coping, ineffective individual; related to manipulation of others	The patient will: • express feelings of anger and frustration verbally rather than by acting out. • identify expectations of others in a relationship. • distinguish between realistic and unrealistic expectations.
Nursing interventions	**Discharge planning**
• Observe how the patient interacts with others. • Provide short, simple explanations of rules and consequences; don't argue with the patient. • Point out any manipulative behaviors and reinforce positive, nonmanipulative behaviors. • Provide a safe therapeutic environment and set limits as needed. • Encourage the patient to explore his feelings and discuss his expectations of the therapeutic relationship. • Demonstrate the difference between realistic and unrealistic expectations, using role-playing.	• Review the patient's care plan with him and his family. • Consult with a psychiatric clinical specialist or community health nurse to provide follow-up care as needed. • Refer the patient and his family to a community self-help group or a treatment center specializing in antisocial personality disorder.

• coping, ineffective individual; related to manipulation of others
• communication, impaired verbal; related to inappropriate expression of anger and hostility
• social isolation; related to manipulative behavior
• sexual dysfunction; related to inability to develop a close and warm relationship with sexual partner
• social interaction, impaired; related to inability to develop and sustain a close and warm relationship
• violence, potential for; related to impulsiveness and acting out.

The sample nursing care plan above shows expected outcomes, nursing interventions, and discharge planning for one of the nursing diagnoses listed above. However, you'll want to individualize your care plan to meet the needs of your patient and his family.

Intervention

Treatment for antisocial personality disorder usually resembles that used for other personality disorders.

Psychodynamic approaches focus on altering personality structure. They involve:
• recognizing how a patient's maladaptive traits are manifested both within and outside of his relationship with his therapist
• tracing the development of maladaptive traits and their connection with family relationships
• providing insight into the unconscious conflicts that underlie these traits.

Treatments methods range from short-term psychotherapy to psychoanalysis conducted several times a week for several years. Usually, treatment doesn't attempt to effect any fundamental change in the patient's personality. Instead, it tries to reduce the inflexibility of his behavior and the adverse effects of his condition on daily function and interpersonal relationships.

Continued on page 136

Personality Disorders

Setting limits effectively

In a therapeutic setting, placing limits on behavior gives the patient a sense of security and self-control, and communicates caring on the part of the staff. Limits help you establish boundaries, such as that the patient may not hurt others or destroy property. They help you to avoid becoming angry and frustrated with the patient, increasing the effectiveness of the therapeutic relationship. The patient will benefit from developing a sense of responsibility for his actions. Use the following guidelines for setting limits effectively:
• Make it clear to the patient what you expect from him. Apply rules consistently and, when possible, offer alternatives to unacceptable behavior.
• Establish limits strictly for the patient's behavior, not for his feelings. Convey that although you don't accept his behavior, you accept him as an individual. If you focus on feelings—such as anger—the patient will sense that his emotions are unacceptable.
• Allow the patient to express his feelings about what limits mean to him. He may perceive them as a message that you no longer like him, or may feel increased anxiety because he isn't used to such external controls.
• Avoid using limits as punishment or retaliation. Don't set limits only when angry or under stress, as this will hurt your efforts to build a therapeutic relationship with the patient.
• Set limits when you first sense that the patient is violating another person's rights. Don't tolerate his behavior for several days and then launch an angry tirade.
• Inform other staff members of your actions. Failing to do so may enable a manipulative patient to split the staff into factions that he can pit against each other.
• Use the same principles when setting limits for an assaultive patient. If you sense the patient is losing control, step in immediately.
• Apply these principles when working with the patient's family. Often, the patient comes from a family that has had little success in establishing discipline. Explain to them that rules may be enforced in a way that communicates love, caring, and acceptance.

Antisocial personality disorder—*continued*

Psychotherapy often revolves around the relationship between patient and therapist. Typically, the patient tends to evoke complementary responses in others; for example, a threatening patient may cause others to become anxious and fearful. Unfortunately, this usually reinforces the patient's intimidating behavior. To counter this destructive pattern, the therapist may adopt a more flexible interpersonal style that in turn encourages a more flexible response in the patient.

Supportive psychotherapy may be used to help the patient through times of stress with the goal of minimizing regression and promoting compliance with treatment. Group and family therapy may also be beneficial. Group therapy may help the patient recognize how his maladaptive personality traits affect others. Family therapy may be needed if family members reinforce the patient's maladaptive traits and impede positive change.

Behavioral therapies, such as shaping (reinforcing responses that resemble sought-after behavior), reinforcement (strengthening response by reward or avoidance of punishment), and systemic desensitization, may prove helpful, especially when focused on a prominent characteristic of the disorder, such as persistent disregard for other's feelings. Cognitive techniques may also prove helpful in addressing irrational thought patterns.

Drug therapy may be used to treat target symptoms or prominent features of the disorder. If the patient's symptoms have a biochemical basis, certain drugs may provide relief. Even if he doesn't have any biochemical abnormalities, drug therapy often helps alleviate symptoms and enhances response to psychotherapy.

Whether *inpatient therapy* should be used remains controversial. Proponents point out the benefits of having the patient in a controlled environment where he can't refuse treatment. Opponents contend that the patient may prevent staff from giving other patients needed attention because he's so demanding and manipulative. His antisocial behavior may force staff to make rules that restrict all patients. Maintaining a therapeutic milieu may require great effort.

Nursing care measures. The patient may express anger and hostility by cursing, screaming, making threats or intimidating gestures, slamming doors, or throwing objects. Clearly explain the consequences of inappropriate displays of anger and hostility.

Setting limits. Until the patient learns to control destructive behavior, you must set limits to discourage such behavior and provide safe boundaries for testing new behaviors. (See *Setting limits effectively.*)

Assess the patient's potential for violence toward himself or others. If his anger seems out of control or on the verge of leading to violence, take the following steps:
• Provide feedback on the patient's nonverbal behavior to help him identify his angry feelings. For example, you might say "You look angry. Can you tell me what you're feeling?"
• Encourage him to express anger in a way that doesn't threaten others. Help him explore alternative methods of expressing aggression, such as punching a pillow or pounding modeling clay.

Personality Disorders

Patients who provoke strong feelings

Patients with antisocial personality disorder frequently act in ways that are likely to provoke strong emotional reactions from you. Be aware of how personal feelings can affect the quality of care.

A threatening patient, for example, may make you fearful, causing you to avoid him. A patient who acts out his sexual feelings by pinching you or exposing himself may become repulsive to you. A seductive patient may evoke various responses, ranging from pleasure to fear, depending upon your own attitude and the individual patient.

For all of these patients, you'll need to set appropriate limits. If you feel threatened by a sexually aggressive patient, ask yourself "What am I afraid this patient would actually do?" The answer will help you identify what restrictions need to be set on the patient's behavior.

Be careful not to set limits that are so harsh they convey to the patient the message that he should be ashamed of his feelings. On the other hand, don't dismiss seductive behavior just because the patient doesn't appear sexually threatening.

When possible, provide honest feedback in a nonpunitive manner. For example, you might say "I feel uncomfortable when you mention overpowering me and I can't allow it to continue. Why do you want to threaten me?" Remember that persistent seductive behavior expresses an underlying need that will have to be addressed.

• Help him explore the source of his anger.
• Take all threats seriously, and prepare to act to maintain a safe environment.
• Determine the need for medication and physical restraints, and notify the doctor as needed.

Battling manipulative behavior. The antisocial patient often uses others to achieve his own ends. He may be skilled at recognizing an individual's weaknesses and exploiting them. Such a patient may easily provoke your anger; you may think he has used you and repaid your concern with ingratitude. Keep in mind the following measures when caring for a manipulative patient:
• Closely observe how he interacts with others. Identify other patients or staff members who could be easily manipulated by him.
• Make expectations and rules clear and set limits when needed. Avoid arguing with the patient. Don't try to convince him your actions are justified. He needs to understand what will and will not be tolerated.
• Review special requests made by the patient with other staff before granting them. Schedule staff conferences to discuss necessary limit setting. Encourage consistent application of rules throughout all shifts.
• Point out manipulative behavior when it occurs and explain to the patient clearly why his actions are unacceptable. Remember that he might not be aware what actions are inappropriate. For example, explain that it's wrong for him to take advantage of people who are afraid to say no to him.
• Help the patient identify his needs and develop alternative ways of coping. This will allow him to feel more in control. Pay attention to him when he's not manipulating others; this will help reinforce positive behavior.

Easing isolation. If the patient appears to retreat from social interaction, encourage him to express his needs and explore together the meaning of his social isolation. Provide positive feedback when he interacts with others appropriately and encourage him to engage in organized group activities. (See *Patients who provoke strong feelings* and *Tips for dealing with antisocial patients,* page 138.)

Evaluation
Base your evaluation on the expected outcomes listed in the nursing care plan. To determine if the patient's improved, ask yourself questions like these:
• Is the patient appropriately expressing anger and frustration?
• Does he understand the expectations of others when entering a relationship?
• Can he distinguish between realistic and unrealistic expectations?

The answers to these questions will help you evaluate the patient's status and the effectiveness of his care. Keep in mind that these questions stem from the sample care plan shown on page 135. Your questions may differ.

Continued on page 138

Personality Disorders

Borderline personality disorder

The patient with borderline personality disorder suffers from a weak self-image. He may be uncertain about long-term goals, sexual orientation, choice of friends, or what values to live by. He may experience intense mood swings and an underlying sense of emptiness or boredom. Because he's unable to develop a cohesive sense of self, he can't form healthy relationships with others. His friendships tend to be intense and erratic. He may be unable to control anger or impulses and behave in self-destructive and self-defeating ways. He may frustrate the staff by crying out for help and then rejecting it when offered.

The affected patient—more commonly female than male—stands out in a hospital setting because of the disorder's chronicity and severity. The disorder itself appears to originate during early childhood. As a toddler, each child needs to establish an identity separate from his parents, realizing that this separation doesn't mean abandonment. Parents can encourage this independence by:
• allowing the child to make minor decisions and helping him in the process when necessary
• making it clear to the child that they accept his feelings but that he must learn to control his impulsive behavior (for example, "We understand you're angry, but you're not allowed to hit your sister.")
• providing clear-cut and consistent rules
• helping the child learn to express his feelings verbally, rather than through impulsive acting out
• helping him integrate positive and negative qualities into a whole identity. Parents may accomplish this by appropriately expressing both positive and negative feelings toward the child (for example, "We love you, but we don't like it when you throw a temper tantrum").

Parents, however, may respond inappropriately to a child's early efforts at independence, increasing his chances of developing borderline personality disorder. For example, they may withdraw approval when their child makes independent decisions, thwarting development. They may perceive autonomous behavior as a threat to family authority and attempt to manipulate the child's feelings; they may say, for instance, "We're going to give you away if you keep acting like this." At the same time, they may reinforce submissive behavior. This behavior pattern may lead to various problems, including:
• a confused sense of self. The child fails to develop an identity apart from his parents or confidence in his ability to function without them. Separation from his parents, even for a short time, evokes severe anxiety and depression.
• an inability to express his feelings adequately. The child may resort to impulsive, acting-out behavior.
• use of defense mechanisms, such as denial and projection. (See *How borderline patients cope.*)

If a child fails to begin to develop his own identity, he'll have increased difficulty in adolescence achieving independence from his

Personality Disorders

How borderline patients cope

Borderline patients rely on the following defense mechanisms to cope with anxiety:

Denial
This defense mechanism represents an unconscious attempt to avoid unacceptable or threatening feelings. Because the patient can't express his feelings adequately, he may act them out through drug abuse, promiscuity, overeating, and other self-destructive acts.

Splitting
Splitting refers to an inability to accept that good and bad qualities can exist in the same individual. The patient views himself and others as all good or all bad. Associated defense mechanisms include idealization—a tendency to idealize individuals perceived as all good—and devaluation—a tendency to devalue others and blame them indiscriminately. When an idealized individual disappoints him, the patient will blame others, blame himself (and punish himself through self-destructive behavior), or devalue the idealized individual.

Projection
In this defense mechanism, the patient unconsciously attempts to project onto others unacceptable qualities in himself. He may blame others for his actions and perceive himself as a victim, powerless to control his own life.

Fostering a healthy sense of individuality

The diagram below outlines the steps of the *separation-individuation* process, whereby the child develops a sense of identity separate from his parents. Healthy passage through this process leads to a strong sense of individuality and self-confidence, whereas a maladaptive response may lead to a weak identity and poor self-esteem. The significance of these issues is not limited to childhood. For example, when the time comes for a therapeutic relationship to end, problems associated with establishing independence that the patient first encountered during childhood may recur. To foster a stronger sense of identity in such a patient, use the same principles—such as consistent limit setting and emotional support—that foster independence during childhood.

	Normal development	Maladaptive response
THE PARENTS:	• allow their child some freedom but remain available and supportive • set limits while allowing freedom within these limits • maintain consistent limits • accept the child's emerging individuality.	• withdraw approval from child when he attempts to separate from the family • set no consistent limits • reject the child's attempts to express his individuality.
THE CHILD:	• develops a sense of individuality • learns to accept and integrate positive and negative aspects of his personality • develops a sense of inner control and discipline.	• loses interest in developing a separate identity • fails to develop self-esteem • perceives himself as bad when he provokes disapproval and good when he can gain approval • engages in impulsive acting-out behavior.

family and developing healthful relationships with peers and the opposite sex. (See *Fostering a healthy sense of individuality.*)

Assessment
To assess for borderline personality disorder, explore the patient's self-esteem and sense of identity. Ask him to describe himself and list his strengths and limitations. How does he act when he feels good about himself? When he feels badly about himself?

Assess the quality of the patient's interpersonal relationships. Ask him to give you his definition of a friend and to describe the individuals he calls friends. Is he able to confide in them? Does he seem to idealize them? Does he devalue other acquaintances? How does he respond if his friends do something he considers wrong or if they refuse to do what he wants?

Assess the patient's family relationships. Is he especially close with any of his relatives? Does he argue with family members? If so, ask him to describe how he reacts during an argument. If he lives with his family, ask if he makes any decisions in his family and to describe his responsibilities.

Find out if the patient is bothered by being alone. Many borderline personality patients will make frantic efforts to avoid abandonment, whether real or imagined.

Assess for unstable affect. The patient may become depressed, irritable, or anxious; mood swings may last from a few hours to a

Continued on page 140

Personality Disorders

Encouraging the patient to express himself

Use the following techniques to encourage the patient with a personality disorder to express his feelings.

Sharing observations
"I notice that you've been sitting with your fists clenched. Are you feeling angry and frustrated?"

Focusing
"When I ask how you feel, you tell me what happened during group therapy yesterday. I'd also like to know how you feel right now."

Verbalizing the implied
"You say that after your father visits you feel like slamming doors and throwing things. Perhaps you do that instead of telling your father you're angry with him because you're afraid that he'd abandon you."

Validating the patient's feelings
"You look angry; can you tell me if that's how you feel?"

Borderline personality disorder—*continued*

few days. He also may display intense anger or lack of control over anger, possibly leading to tantrums. Ask if he frequently gets into fights. Also assess for impulsive behavior, such as shopping sprees, drug and alcohol abuse, vandalism, reckless driving, promiscuous sex, shoplifting, and binge eating. Remember that for the patient these destructive behaviors represent a way of acting out anger, frustration, and anxiety.

Gauge the risk of self-destructive behavior in patients with severe forms of the disorder. Such patients may make repeated suicidal threats or attempts. They may mutilate themselves as a means to manipulate others, express anger, or fight feelings of numbness and depersonalization.

Intervention

The patient may benefit from psychotherapy. In individual psychotherapy, though, the patient's relationship with the therapist can become too intense. As a result, group or family therapy may be preferable. Cognitive therapeutic techniques may help him confront his tendency to idealize or devalue others and develop more realistic perceptions.

Various drug therapies have been used to treat borderline personality disorder, with varying success. Because of the disorder's somewhat nebulous nature, doctors usually focus on treating the patient's major symptoms rather than rely on a predetermined regimen. For example, a patient with distorted cognition may benefit from a neuroleptic. A patient suffering from mood swings may get relief from lithium, while a patient with intense dysphoria may require monoamine oxidase inhibitor therapy.

A patient with borderline personality disorder often causes serious stress on a medical-surgical unit, partly because of his tendency to idolize some staff members and devalue others. Divisiveness, anger, and discouragement among staff may lead to deterioration in the patient's condition, especially if frustrated staff members reject the patient or lose their ability to deal with him effectively. Conflicts may occur if the patient is out of touch with the staff's perception of reality, becomes overly aggressive, or seeks too much personal closeness.

Consultation with a staff psychiatrist may help reduce conflict. Besides helping with patient diagnosis and treatment, a psychiatric consultant can monitor stress among staff members and help them develop and improve strategies for dealing with the patient.

Nursing care measures. These measures include providing a safe and therapeutic environment to help the patient develop effective coping strategies and increase self-esteem. This means showing support and acceptance as he tests new behaviors and setting consistent limits to decrease acting-out behavior.

Use effective communication techniques, such as sharing observations and verbalizing what the patient implies. (See *Encouraging the patient to express himself.*) In both one-to-one and group therapy situations, encourage him to express himself. If you wait for him

Personality Disorders

Overcoming barriers with the borderline patient

When caring for the borderline personality patient, keep in mind that he may devalue and manipulate you and others to protect himself from the anxiety associated with interpersonal relationships. Even if you have considerable self-esteem and confidence, you may become frustrated at his lack of progress. You may even project your own unresolved emotional conflicts onto the patient (countertransference). Such reactions may cause you to avoid the patient or become locked in a power struggle with him. To avoid this, carefully assess your own feelings. Ask yourself these questions:
• How do I view myself? Do I accept both my good and my bad qualities?
• What can I accept and not accept in others?
• How do I deal with sadness, anger, boredom, loneliness, emptiness, and frustration?
• How do I cope with difficulties in relationships?
• Do I devalue others so I can feel better about myself?

Consulting with a psychiatric liaison nurse, a psychiatric clinical specialist, or psychiatrist may help you learn the answers to these questions and improve your relationship with the borderline personality patient.

to initiate the discussion, very little may happen. Avoid such judgmental statements as "You shouldn't feel annoyed." Be aware of your body language, such as frowning or pulling back when the patient becomes angry.

If the patient won't or can't discuss his feelings, encourage some other form of communication, such as keeping and sharing a diary, creating artwork, or sharing a piece of music that expresses an important emotion.

Try to help improve the patient's self-esteem. Help him learn to accept his positive and negative qualities. Telling him to accept himself isn't enough; you need to demonstrate acceptance during both good and bad times. For example, instead of telling the patient that you won't talk to him until he "shapes up"—a message that he'll perceive as rejection—give him the opportunity to decide for himself how he should behave. If he acts inappropriately, don't criticize; instead, explain that he'll get other chances to behave better and help him explore the meaning of his behavior.

Instilling in the patient a sense of control over his environment will help him develop confidence in his decision-making ability. Your approach will depend on the patient's anxiety level. A patient with low self-esteem and a high anxiety level may need you to temporarily make most decisions. As his anxiety diminishes, allow him to make more complex decisions. Continue to support him and help him understand the consequences of each decision. (See *Overcoming barriers with the borderline patient.*)

Self-test

1. A general profile of the substance abuse patient might include all of the following, except:
a. Outwardly he appears domineering but inwardly he feels passive **b.** He uses defense mechanisms to justify behavior **c.** Because of guilt, he eagerly makes confessions about his drug habit **d.** He manipulates others to obtain his drug of choice

2. Potential effects of alcohol abuse include all of the following except:
a. loss of remote memory with retention of short-term memory **b.** increased hostility or aggressiveness **c.** peripheral neuropathy, cardiomyopathy, and sexual dysfunction **d.** cancer

3. Which of the following treatments for antisocial patients is the most controversial?
a. individual psychotherapy **b.** behavioral therapy **c.** drug therapy targeted to specific symptoms **d.** inpatient therapy

4. When setting limits, allow a patient who acts destructively to vent his aggressions and see if he regains self-control on his own before stepping in.
a. true **b.** false

Answers (page number shows where answer appears in text)
1. **c** (page 111)   2. **a** (page 119)   3. **d** (page 136)   4. **b** (page 136)

Organic Mental Disorders: Alzheimer's Disease and Other Dementias

Jill Shapira, the author of this chapter, is a clinical nurse specialist at West Los Angeles Veterans Administration Medical Center's Brentwood Division. She earned her BS and MN from the University of California at Los Angeles.

All organic mental disorders share one common feature: an abnormal mental status caused by brain dysfunction. This dysfunction commonly causes confusion, memory loss, and language difficulties.

Organic mental disorders may arise from various causes, including:
• primary disease of the brain, such as Alzheimer's disease
• a physical disorder, such as neurosyphilis, that causes a secondary brain disease
• abuse of alcohol, psychoactive drugs, or toxic agents
• withdrawal from a psychoactive substance
• brain injury from head trauma.
See *Causes of organic mental disorders* for further information.

The course of these disorders differs considerably. For example, Alzheimer's patients grow progressively worse over 8 to 12 years and eventually die, while patients with delirium develop symptoms suddenly and may recover completely if the underlying condition receives proper treatment. (See *Dealing with delirium.*)

In this chapter, we'll focus on assessment and intervention for the major dementias. Dementias affect elderly persons most often; an estimated 5% of elderly persons suffer severe intellectual impairment due to dementia, and 10% to 15% suffer mild to moderate impairment.

Causes of organic mental disorders

Organic mental disorders can result from extrapyramidal conditions, central nervous system (CNS) disturbances, systemic illnesses, endocrine disturbances, and deficiency states.

Extrapyramidal conditions
• Huntington's disease
• Parkinson's disease

CNS disturbances
• Alzheimer's disease
• Cerebrovascular disease
• Epilepsy
• Meningitis
• Multiple sclerosis
• Neoplasms
• Syphilis
• Viral encephalitis

Systemic illness
• Anoxia
• Hepatic encephalopathy
• Hypercalcemia
• Hypoglycemia
• Hyponatremia
• Pancreatic encephalopathy
• Subacute bacterial endocarditis
• Uremia

Endocrine diseases
• Addison's disease
• Cushing's disease
• Diabetic ketoacidosis
• Hyperthyroidism
• Hypothyroidism

Deficiency states
• Folate
• Niacin
• Thiamine
• Vitamin B_{12}

Dementias

Dementia refers to an acquired, chronic loss of intellectual function that affects at least three areas of mental activity. Affected areas may include memory, language, visuospatial skills, motor function, and cognition. Impaired intellectual activity commonly leads to marked changes in affect and personality. Major types of dementia include:
• Alzheimer's disease
• pseudodementia
• multi-infarct dementia
• extrapyramidal disorders
• chronic confusional states.

Alzheimer's disease. Accounting for 40% to 60% of all irreversible dementias, Alzheimer's disease develops insidiously, with its risk increasing with age. Overt symptoms usually appear after age 55. The disease strikes equal numbers of men and women.

Alzheimer's disease is characterized by reduced levels of choline acetyltransferase, the enzyme that synthesizes acetylcholine in the brain. This reduction causes a loss of neurons in the cortical area, along with characteristic neurofibrillary tangles and senile plaques. Steady, progressive intellectual deterioration occurs in three stages without remission. (See *What causes Alzheimer's disease?*, page 144.)

Early stage. The patient will usually first experience amnesia. He may have difficulty recalling new information, such as the date or the content of a recent conversation. He may rationalize his diminishing memory by saying "I was never good with dates" or "I could never keep up with current events."

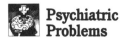
Organic Mental Disorders

The patient may also have trouble recalling remote information, such as early life events or historical facts. Typically, he'll appear apathetic toward his memory difficulties or deny them.

Although the patient's lip and tongue muscles aren't impaired, aphasia may occur. He may grope for words when speaking extemporaneously. He may have trouble naming objects in a specific category, such as animals, cities, or articles of clothing (anomia), or comprehending other people's speech.

The patient's visuospatial skills may become impaired. For example, he may lose his way when walking in familiar surroundings or when driving. This often causes family members to realize his problem is more severe than mere forgetfulness.

Signs of cognitive impairment may include a progressive decline in computation skills and poor reason and judgment. The patient may

Continued on page 144

Dealing with delirium

Delirium refers to a rapid behavior change marked by decreased attention span, disorganized thinking, incoherency, and rambling, irrelevant speech. Up to 15% of medical-surgical unit patients develop delirium during hospitalization; among elderly patients, the figure rises to 40%.

Signs and symptoms

Onset is acute and signs and symptoms may fluctuate over the course of a day, with confusion usually increasing at night (sundown syndrome). Each episode of delirium usually lasts for a few hours or days. However, delirium may last for weeks in elderly patients.

An impaired level of awareness may lead to attention deficits and an increased susceptibility to distraction. Attention deficits, in turn, may impair the patient's memory, and he may become disoriented to time, date, and place. In addition, he may become confused about recent events. For example, he may claim he has just seen a movie when he's actually been in the X-ray department all day. He may also misname familiar objects, making it difficult to follow his conversation.

The patient may also experience nighttime restlessness and daytime drowsiness or visual, auditory, or tactile hallucinations. When agitated, he may pull out catheters or I.V. lines and, in general, match the textbook description of a confused patient. However, his behavior can also be just the opposite: he may become hypoactive or even stuporous, drifting in and out of consciousness.

Neurologic signs associated with delirium include postural or action tremors, sudden and unsustained muscle contractions (myoclonus), flapping tremors (asterixis), and slurred speech.

Causes

Possible causes of delirium include cardiovascular, central nervous system, and metabolic disorders as well as such conditions as systemic infection and trauma. Elderly patients are especially susceptible to delirium caused by metabolic change, infection, or drug toxicity or withdrawal effects.

Diagnosis

Because delirium can be treated, distinguishing it from Alzheimer's disease is crucial. Remember

that delirium develops abruptly and attention deficit impairs memory, whereas Alzheimer's begins insidiously and memory is actually lost. What's more, the patient with delirium is more likely to have a history of systemic illness or exposure to toxic substances. And while EEG studies of the Alzheimer's patient are unremarkable, EEGs of the patient with delirium show pronounced diffuse slowing.

Keep in mind, though, that patients with Alzheimer's disease, multi-infarct dementia, and other dementias may develop infections that can lead to superimposed delirium.

Intervention

Report any signs of delirium to the doctor immediately. Treatment may include low doses of a major tranquilizer, such as haloperidol (Haldol). Work with the health care team to correct the underlying cause of delirium.

Help the patient become oriented by hanging a calendar on his wall and by providing a clock, television, and radio. Encourage family members to bring familiar items and photographs and to visit the patient often. Reassure them that you expect the patient to improve with treatment.

When approaching the patient, identify yourself as a nurse and explain what you plan to do, using short, direct statements. You may communicate better by referring to his experiences or interests, perhaps mentioning children or grandchildren, pets, or his occupation.

If the patient becomes hostile, he probably senses a threat to his safety. Calmly say to him, "I know you feel afraid, but I won't hurt you. I'm here to help you."

If the patient pulls out his catheter or I.V. or tries to remove his dressings, you may have to put mittens on him or apply restraints. Tell him that you're restraining him for his own safety and that you understand how upset he feels. Explain to his family you'll remove the restraints once delirium abates.

Organic Mental Disorders

What causes Alzheimer's disease?

Scientists still don't know the cause of Alzheimer's disease. However, they've put forth several possible explanations.

Aluminum toxicity
Rabbits exposed to toxic amounts of aluminum develop neurofibrillary tangles, suggesting aluminum poisoning may cause Alzheimer's disease. However, these tangles differ from those of Alzheimer's patients, and patients don't show elevated aluminum levels in their blood or cerebrospinal fluid.

Serum protein abnormalities
Found in some Alzheimer's patients, serum protein abnormalities suggest that the disease might result from an immunologic dysfunction. However, these abnormalities may occur secondary to some other process.

Viruses
Researchers have suggested a viral cause for Alzheimer's disease. However, efforts to transmit Alzheimer's disease by inoculating laboratory animals with brain tissue of affected patients have failed.

Nerve cell defects
Cellular abnormalities in Alzheimer's disease resemble those in Down's syndrome and hematologic disorders, providing the basis for this theory.

Genetic predisposition
Genetic inheritance offers the most likely explanation of Alzheimer's disease. Offspring of Alzheimer's patients face an increased risk of acquiring the disease. In addition, patients are more likely to have a family history of Down's syndrome, hematologic cancers, and abnormalities of lymphocyte chromosomes than the general population.

Dementias—*continued*

make unwise business decisions or errors when filling out income tax forms or balancing his checkbook.

The patient may also lose the ability to act spontaneously or become disinterested in his hobbies. Occasionally, he may experience depression during the early stage of illness. As symptoms worsen, depression will disappear.

Despite intellectual deterioration, the patient's social skills often remain largely intact. A patient with severe memory or cognitive impairment may continue to function until a change in circumstances or new demands make it impossible for him to hide his dementia.

Middle stage. At this point, spatial comprehension may deteriorate drastically, and the patient may have trouble dressing himself. He may exhibit restlessness, pacing, outbursts of temper, or sudden, unprovoked crying. He may develop suspicious delusions, believing that his spouse is unfaithful or that a stranger is living in his home and stealing things. Language disturbances increase; the patient may become incomprehensible or mute. Eventually, he ceases to recognize his home or family members. He may even cease to recognize himself in the mirror and begin to talk to his reflection. Typically, he becomes incontinent. Motor function usually remains unaffected until the late stage of illness.

Late stage. In this stage, muscles become rigid and flexed. Such primitive reflexes as grasping and sucking predominate, and the patient usually assumes the fetal position. Seizures, while not common, may occur during this stage. Death usually occurs from aspiration pneumonia, urinary tract infection, or infection of decubitus ulcers.

Pseudodementia. Also called dementia syndrome of depression, pseudodementia refers to a reversible, functional condition resembling and frequently misdiagnosed as Alzheimer's disease. Distinguishing between the two is important because antidepressant drugs may reverse the forgetfulness, withdrawal, disorientation, and confusion that occurs in pseudodementia. Unfortunately, patients with pseudodementia do not visit a doctor until their symptoms becomes so severe that their condition is almost indistinguishable from Alzheimer's disease.

Sometimes trial treatment with antidepressant drugs offers the only means to differentiate pseudodementia from Alzheimer's disease or, if both disorders coexist, to determine the relative impact of each. For example, after taking antidepressants, a patient with pseudodementia may experience dramatic cognitive improvement whereas an Alzheimer's patient would not.

Multi-infarct dementia (MID). The second most common dementia, MID results from multiple vascular strokes. The disorder most often occurs between ages 50 to 70, and its course from onset to death usually takes 5 to 8 years.

Signs of MID depend on the location and amount of infarcted tissue. (See *Multi-infarct dementia.*) The patient usually exhibits abrupt behavioral changes, though his overall personality may remain

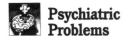
Organic Mental Disorders

Multi-infarct dementia

The illustration below depicts a posterior view of the cerebrum of a patient with multi-infarct dementia (MID). Tissue necrosis, indicated by the darkened areas, appears in the parietal lobe. This necrosis may lead to sensory difficulties, problems with body integration, and loss of two- and three-point discrimination.

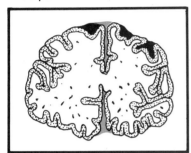

relatively stable. Other symptoms include depression, emotional lability, and inappropriate affect. The patient experiences a stepwise decline in intellectual function, with multiple remissions. His condition worsens with each new stroke.

The MID patient may have a history of hypertension, cerebrovascular accident, diabetes, inflammatory disease, embolytic disorders, or atherosclerosis outside of the brain. He may display focal neurologic signs or bilateral abnormalities including rigidity, spasticity, hyperreflexia, extensor plantar responses, and gait abnormalities.

Extrapyramidal disorders. These dementias affect the subcortical structures (basal ganglia, thalamus, and brainstem) and produce symptoms distinct from Alzheimer's disease (which generally affects the cerebral cortex). The most common subcortical dementias are Parkinson's disease and Huntington's disease; less common ones include Wilson's disease, progressive supranuclear palsy, spinocerebellar degeneration, and idiopathic basal ganglia calcification.

Affected patients experience depression as part of their disease, not simply as a response to physical disability. They also experience depression more frequently than patients with other chronic neurologic conditions. Other symptoms include forgetfulness; cognitive slowness; movement disorders, such as chorea and tremors; muscle rigidity; and speech articulation problems (dysarthria).

Parkinson's disease. The neurologic disorder most commonly associated with aging, Parkinson's disease characteristically develops between ages 50 and 65, striking more men than women. Its course averages 8 years, with death resulting from aspiration pneumonia, urinary tract infection, or unrelated disorders.

Lack of dopamine, a neurotransmitter normally found in the basal ganglia, causes Parkinson's disease. The disorder is slowly progressive and symptoms include bradykinesia, cogwheel rigidity, resting tremor, masked facies, excessive perspiration, drooling, and gait, posture, and equilibrium disturbances. (See *Selected signs of Parkinson's disease*, page 146.)

Huntington's disease. This idiopathic, degenerative disease usually appears between ages 35 and 40 and lasts about 15 years. Inherited as an autosomal dominant pattern, it strikes 50% of the offspring of affected individuals and is equally common in men and women. Death most commonly results from aspiration pneumonia or urinary tract infection.

Huntington's disease causes marked cell loss in the basal ganglia, especially the caudate nucleus. Along with dementia, the patient experiences chorea, with facial grimacing, head nodding, truncal and limb jerks, and flexion-extension movements of the fingers.

Chronic confusional states. These states may result from metabolic or toxic encephalopathies or from increased intracranial pressure. When a metabolic disturbance or toxic exposure occurs gradually, dementia progresses slowly. The patient experiences symptoms similar to those caused by impaired subcortical function, including psychomotor slowing, memory loss, attention disturbances, and mood changes.

Continued on page 146

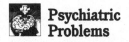
Organic Mental Disorders

Dementias—*continued*

Metabolic encephalopathies. Dementias from these encephalopathies occur primarily in elderly patients. They may stem from chronic conditions that affect cerebral function, such as cardiac or hepatic failure, pulmonary insufficiency, or renal disease. Dementias may also result from endocrine disorders (especially in the thyroid, parathyroid, and adrenal glands); vitamin B_{12}, folate, or niacin deficiencies; organisms that directly invade the brain (such as the human immunodeficiency virus); or neurosyphilis, chronic meningitis, or Jakob-Creutzfeldt disease.

Toxic encephalopathies. These encephalopathies may occur with use of psychotropic agents, antihypertensives, anticonvulsants, digitalis, and other drugs. Chronic drug or alcohol abuse may also cause dementias that frequently improve or disappear after withdrawal.

Industrial agents, such as organic solvents and heavy metals, can also impair neurologic function and cause toxic encephalopathies. Such substances may impair both central and peripheral nervous system tissues, leading to peripheral neuropathies. Patients may experience decreased sensation in their hands and feet, causing gait disturbances and increasing the risk of serious falls as well as skin ulcerations or burns from injury or hot water.

Increased intracranial pressure. Cerebral neoplasms and subdural hematomas represent the chief causes of increased intracranial pressure leading to chronic confusional states. In patients with intracranial tumors, symptoms of dementia depend upon the lesion's location.

Doctors often mistakenly diagnose subdural hematoma as Alzheimer's disease or MID—possibly delaying surgical treatment. In elderly patients, the most common symptoms of subdural hematoma include fluctuating arousal, poor attention span, irritability, and memory loss. Patients may have experienced minimal serious head trauma or none at all.

Assessment

Assessing for an organic mental disorder includes taking a patient history, interviewing family members, performing physical and neurologic examinations, testing mental status, and obtaining necessary diagnostic studies.

Patient history. When taking the history, focus on changes in the patient's behavior. Ask about recent memory loss or communication problems. Does the patient frequently get lost in familiar surroundings? What tasks can he accomplish today compared to what he could do 6 to 12 months ago? Ask about past systemic illness or exposure to toxic substances. If the patient's confused, ask family members for clarification. Also ask them if the patient's social behavior is frequently inappropriate. (See *Assessing dementia: Taking a patient history.*)

Take a careful medication history, asking about use of over-the-counter and illicit drugs. Pay special attention to whether changes in medications or dosages coincide with onset of symptoms. Is the patient relying too heavily on any particular drugs? Is he taking

Selected signs of Parkinson's disease

Motor disturbances, such as muscle rigidity, akinesia, and involuntary tremor, constitute the cardinal symptoms of Parkinson's disease. Proper assessment requires identifying characteristic signs and symptoms, such as those illustrated below:

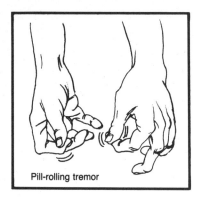

Pill-rolling tremor

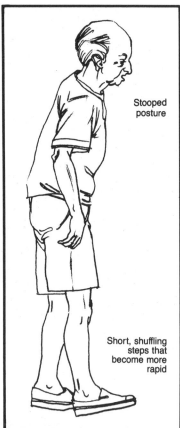

Stooped posture

Short, shuffling steps that become more rapid

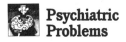
Organic Mental Disorders

When assessing a patient for dementia, you'll need to determine the answers to these questions.

☐ Does he complain of memory loss or memory deficit?
☐ Does he complain of forgetting the location of familiar objects or forgetting familiar names?
☐ How concerned is he about memory loss?
☐ Are others, such as family members and employers, aware of the patient's memory lapses?
☐ Has he lost the ability to recall the content of a story, either read or heard?
☐ Does he try to hide signs of impaired mentation?
☐ Do neuropsychiatric examination results show evidence of memory and concentration deficits?
☐ Can he manage complex tasks?
☐ Has he exhibited lability of affect?
☐ Does he remember telephone numbers, dates of important events, and names of close family members?
☐ Has he become disoriented to time, person, and place?
☐ Have his sleep and wake cycles changed?
☐ Can he hold a conversation or utter meaningful sounds?
☐ Can he perform psychomotor tasks?
☐ Is he incontinent?

any drug that is past its expiration date? Many elderly patients use outdated drugs, which may cause toxicity as a result of pharmacologic changes.

Family history. Ask the patient and his relatives if the family has any history of Down's syndrome, hematologic cancers, vascular disease, dementia, depression, or movement disorders.

Physical and neurologic examination. A general physical examination may reveal a systemic illness, and a detailed neurologic examination may reveal signs of a central nervous system disorder. When performing a neurologic examination, assess the cranial nerves, motor function, sensation, and reflexes. Give a complete description of any movement disorder. Focal findings may indicate lateral brain involvement, such as multiple cerebral infarctions, neoplasm, or subdural hematoma.

Mental status examination. A thorough mental status examination should include tests of attention level, awareness, language skills, memory, visuospatial skills, and cognition. When assessing for dementia, use the mental status examination to:
• assess problems with brain function
• obtain an ongoing assessment of the patient's strengths and weaknesses
• help plan nursing interventions
• determine whether the patient's ready to learn self-care measures.
(See *Assessing cognition quickly,* page 148.)

Attention level. Begin the mental status examination by observing the patient's attention level. Is he able to maintain a coherent line of thought? Is he easily distracted? The rest of your evaluation, of course, depends on the patient's ability to concentrate on the test.

To further evaluate attention level, use the digit span and the "A" test. The digit span measures the ability to focus attention for a short time period. (See Chapter 1 for a description of this test.) To perform the "A" test, recite a series of letters and ask the patient to indicate each time you say the letter "A." If the patient misses any, he may have an attention deficit, a common symptom in dementias caused by toxic and metabolic encephalopathies or increased intracranial pressure, as well as in pseudodementia.

Awareness. Is the patient alert or dull? Wide awake or drowsy? If aroused, can he maintain attention, or does he drift back to sleep? Does his level of awareness change during the interview or in the course of a day?

Language skills. Evaluate these skills. The patient with an organic mental disorder may lose his ability to express himself verbally or in writing or to comprehend spoken or written language.

To assess for aphasia, listen to the patient speak extemporaneously. Is he fluent? Does he stutter, speak extremely softly (hypophonia), or elaborate trivial details (circumstantiality)? Assess his speech comprehension by giving one-step commands (such as "Point to your nose") or three-step commands (such as "Point to the door, the ceiling, and then the floor"). As a more complex test, ask him point to an object you describe (such as "Point to the source of light").

Continued on page 148

Organic Mental Disorders

Assessing cognition quickly

An abbreviated mental status examination offers a practical way to assess a patient's cognitive functioning. The following are sample questions taken from one such examination:

Orientation
1. Ask the patient the year, season, day, and month.
2. Ask him to name the state, county, town, and hospital where he is located.

Registration
3. Say the words "ball," "flag," and "tree" clearly and slowly. Ask the patient to repeat them. Count the number of trials necessary.

Attention and calculation
4. Ask the patient to count backwards by 7, beginning with 100. Stop after 5 subtractions (93, 86, 79, 72, 65). If the patient cannot perform any calculations, use question 5 as a substitute.
5. Tell him to spell the word "world" backward. Award one point for each letter in correct order.

Recall
6. Ask the patient to repeat the three words you had asked him to recite in question 3.

Language
7. Show the patient a wrist watch and a pencil and ask what each one is.
8. Ask him to repeat the phrase "No ifs, ands, or buts."
9. Ask him to follow a three-stage command, such as "Take a piece of paper in your right hand, fold it in half, and put it on the floor."

10. Give him a blank piece of paper and ask him to write a sentence. Check if the sentence makes sense and whether it contains a subject and predicate. Correct grammar and punctuation are less important.

Visual comprehension
11. Ask the patient to copy the design below. Check if all angles are present and if the two shapes intersect.

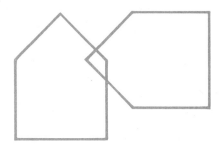

Level of consciousness
12. Assess level of consciousness along the following continuum:

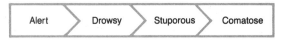

Alert → Drowsy → Stuporous → Comatose

Dementias—*continued*

Ask the patient to name objects you hold up, such as a pencil or a watch. Then have him name parts of each object, such as the eraser or watchband. This seemingly simple task requires use of much of the brain.

Word-list generation. Ask the patient to generate a list of words belonging to a specific category. For example, ask him to name as many different animals as he can think of in 60 seconds. Naming 18 or more animals is considered normal; naming fewer than 12 animals may indicate cortical or subcortical types of dementia.

Writing skills. Tell the patient to write a complete sentence. Then evaluate its content and form. Is it filled with minute, unnecessary detail? Is it repetitious or illegible? Alzheimer's disease and MID disrupt writing skills.

Memory evaluation. Almost all dementias produce memory abnormalities. Evaluate the patient's ability to learn new material (recent memory) by assessing his orientation to time and place. Also, ask him to repeat three unrelated words, wait 3 to 10 minutes (you may perform other tests during this period), and have him repeat these words again. A patient with an organic mental disorder won't be able to recall all three.

To test remote memory, ask the names of past presidents or inquire about memorable political events. Keep in mind that testing remote

Organic Mental Disorders

Diagnostic tests

In a patient with an organic mental disorder, use the following tests to determine the probable cause. Test selection should be based on clinical signs and symptoms.

Test	Implications of abnormal findings
Complete blood count	
Leukocytosis	Infection, mercury toxicity
Lymphocytosis	Mononucleosis, tuberculosis, leukemia
Monocytosis	Brucellosis, rickettsial infection
Leukopenia	Acquired immunodeficiency syndrome, viral encephalitis
Eosinophilia	Parasitic infections, collagen disease
Anemia	Lead toxicity; iron, folate, or B_{12} deficiency
Electrolytes	
Hyponatremia	Addison's disease, water intoxication
Hypernatremia	Diabetes insipidus
Hyperkalemia	Renal or adrenal disease
Hypokalemia	Diuretic use
Hypercalcemia	Hyperparathyroidism
Hypocalcemia	Hypoparathyroidism
Erythrocyte sedimentation rate	Autoimmune disease, infection, neoplasm
Blood glucose	Diabetes, Cushing's disease
Blood urea nitrogen	Renal disease
Creatine phosphokinase	Neuroleptic malignant syndrome
Cholesterol	Thyroid disease, artherosclerosis
Creatinine	Renal disease
Venereal Disease Research Laboratories test	Syphilis, systemic lupus erythematosus
Alkaline phosphatase	Pernicious anemia, scurvy
Drug screen	Alcohol and substance abuse
Thyroid function	Hyperthyroidism, hypothyroidism
Heavy metal screening	Arsenic, mercury, or lead toxicity
Ceruloplasmin	Wilson's disease
Arterial blood gases	Hypoxia, hypercapnia

memory may be difficult because you can't be sure of the patient's past knowledge.

Visuospatial skills. Asking the patient to copy a three-dimensional drawing may provide a sensitive index of cerebral dysfunction. Inability to complete this test often reveals damage to parts of the brain that routine neurologic tests fail to uncover.

Cognition. Assess the patient's ability to use language and memory to manipulate knowledge. A decline in the ability to perform calculations or to think abstractly likely indicates dementia. To test calculation skills, have the patient do simple arithmetic problems. To test ability to understand abstract concepts, first ask him to interpret simple idioms; for example, ask the meaning of "loud" in the sentence "He's wearing a loud tie." Then ask the meaning of proverbs, such as "Don't cry over spilled milk." Literal interpretations of proverbs usually indicate disrupted abstract thinking.

Diagnostic tests. Such studies may help to indicate whether the patient has a treatable condition and may include a complete blood count, erythrocyte sedimentation rate, serum electrolyte and glucose levels, blood urea nitrogen and creatinine levels, serum phosphorus levels, liver and thyroid function tests, serum B_{12} and folate levels, a syphilis test, and a heavy metal and drug screen. (See *Diagnostic tests.*) The doctor may also order an EKG and a chest X-ray to assess cardiopulmonary function.

Continued on page 150

Organic Mental Disorders

Advanced imaging techniques, such as positron emission tomography (PET), are becoming increasingly important in the study of Alzheimer's disease. For example, the PET scan of the brain of an Alzheimer's patient's shows poor glucose use (demonstrated by gaps in the image), whereas the scan of a healthy brain shows ample glucose diffusion.

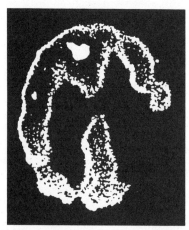

PET scan in Alzheimer's disease

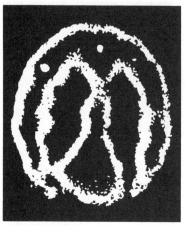

Normal PET scan

Dementias—*continued*

In addition, an EEG can provide important information. A normal tracing suggests that the patient has pseudodementia or has entered the early stages of degenerative dementia. Diffuse EEG slowing may indicate a metabolic or toxic encephalopathy. Focal EEG slowing may indicate a neoplasm, stroke, or subdural hematoma.

Scanning techniques. Computed tomography (CT) scans may help evaluate organic mental disorders, especially focal lesions. However, when no structural changes are evident, their value diminishes. Magnetic resonance imaging (MRI) scans can point out vascular events and show invasive neoplasms. Though not yet widely available, positron emission tomography (PET) scans may reveal poor cerebral glucose use in Alzheimer's disease. (See *Looking at Alzheimer's disease.*) Single-photon emission computed tomography (SPECT) scans may detect regions of poor cerebral perfusion in Alzheimer's disease. Keep in mind, however, that no specific test exists for Alzheimer's disease.

If diagnostic tests indicate the patient has an infection, such as syphilis, the doctor may order a lumbar puncture. The patient may also have to undergo nonspecific tests, such as serum copper, ceruloplasmin, or heavy metal levels, if his history or the physical examination warrants them.

Planning

When planning your care, focus on the patient's physical and safety needs, his psychosocial needs, previous levels of adjustment, and his response to medical and nursing interventions. You'll need to adjust nursing care measures to accommodate the patient's impaired level of understanding. Before writing your nursing care plan, develop the nursing diagnosis by identifying the patient's problem or potential problem, then relating it to its cause. Possible nursing diagnoses for a patient with an organic mental disorder include:

- thought processes, altered; related to brain dysfunction secondary to Alzheimer's disease or MID
- self-care deficit (total); related to memory impairment
- social interaction, impaired; related to language and memory difficulties
- incontinence, functional; related to disease process
- injury, potential for (trauma); related to memory loss
- communication, impaired; related to organic brain dysfunction
- nutrition, altered (less than body requirements); related to forgetting to eat
- mobility, impaired physical; related to specific condition causing gait disturbance
- skin integrity, impaired; related to weight loss and impaired mobility
- infection, potential for; related to impaired skin integrity
- sleep pattern disturbance; related to specific condition
- coping, ineffective family; related to burden of providing care, role changes, financial stress, grieving, and depression.

The sample nursing care plan on the opposite page shows expected outcomes, interventions, and discharge planning for one nursing diagnosis listed above. However, you'll want to individualize your care plan to meet the needs of your patient and his family.

Organic Mental Disorders

Sample nursing care plan: Organic mental disorder

Nursing diagnosis	Expected outcomes
Communication, impaired; related to organic brain dysfunction	The patient will: • be encouraged to communicate at his level of ability. • follow directions when given appropriate cues.

Nursing interventions	Discharge planning
• Initiate and maintain direct eye contact with the patient. • Help him put on eyeglasses or adjust a hearing aid, if appropriate. • Present information in a distraction-free environment. • Give clear, simple, specific directions. • Post important information in the patient's room and bathroom if he can read. Otherwise, post pictures.	• Review the care plan with the patient and his family. • Teach the family effective coping strategies. • Consult with the psychiatric clinical specialist or community nurse to provide follow-up care in the patient's home, as needed. • Refer the patient and his family to a community organization, such as the Alzheimer's Disease and Related Disorders Association.

Intervention

Nursing care measures include protecting the patient from harm, assisting with self-care, preserving the patient's dignity and self-esteem, and supporting the family. With any organic disorder, continually assess for changes in behavior or mental status. Keep in mind that even if the patient suffers from an irreversible dementia, specific behavior changes may have a treatable cause. For example, behavior changes in a patient with Alzheimer's disease may indicate a coexisting urinary tract infection.

Dealing with Alzheimer's disease. Because no treatment can reverse or halt the disease's course, intervention focuses on the patient's behavior.

Communication. Assess the patient's sight and hearing, and assist him with glasses or hearing aids as necessary. If he can't read, help him locate his room by hanging his picture or a picture of his favorite object on the door. To help him understand what he's told, minimize distractions, for example, by turning off television sets and radios.

Observe carefully the patient who can't express himself verbally. If he becomes restless or agitated, for example, he may be in pain or need to use the bathroom. (See *Communicating with Alzheimer's patients*, page 152.)

Providing stimulation. Such activities as puzzles and paint-by-number sets may enable the patient to occupy his time and use his remaining skills. Encourage family members to take walks with the patient. If the patient's bedridden or in the final stages of Alzheimer's disease, maintain proper positioning and perform passive range-of-motion exercises. Provide stimulation by playing soft music, showing him bright pictures, and having him touch objects of varying textures.

Activities of daily living. To help the patient preserve daily living skills, encourage him to care for himself as much as possible. While some patients may initiate self-care, others need help getting started. For example, a patient might not brush his teeth unless you place the toothbrush in his hand. As the disease progresses,

Continued on page 152

Organic Mental Disorders

When speaking to an Alzheimer's patient, be sure to face him, maintain eye contact, and smile. Speak slowly in clear, low tones using simple, direct language. Repeat your remarks as needed.

Use the following tips for establishing nonverbal communication:
• Recognize that the patient may be sensitive to your unspoken feelings about him.
• Shake hands with him if he seems receptive.
• Be aware of what the patient's body language (gestures, facial expressions, and postures) as well as yours conveys.
• Demonstrate your meaning with gestures and actions. For example, point to objects or body parts or act out a concept, such as eating.

expect the patient to become increasingly dependent on others to maintain hygiene.

When helping with hygiene, keep in mind that the patient may easily become agitated; approach him calmly and don't rush him. Note if there's a time of day when the patient's more receptive to help. Orient him by describing the toilet articles you're using, by letting him feel warm running water, and by asking him to stretch his arms before you help him put on clothes. Also, even if he appears oblivious, take measures to protect his right to privacy during self-care activities.

Eating. Provide the patient with a calm, quiet environment during meals. When feeding him, make sure he's sitting upright with his head slightly flexed. Avoid feeding when he's sleepy or agitated. Don't offer foods that he may choke on, such as candy or nuts; provide thick, soft foods instead. To prevent burns, check food temperature. Consider the following guidelines when planning meals:
• Use plastic dishes to avoid injury.
• Use heavy silverware to provide tactile stimulation.
• Offer one food at a time so the patient won't have to make choices.
• Avoid foods of contrasting textures, such as cereal and milk, because the patient may not know whether to chew or swallow.
• Encourage family members or friends to assist at meals.
• Keep between-meal snacks available in case the patient forgets that he's eaten, or to distract him if he becomes agitated.

Monitor food and fluid intake and provide between-meal liquids to maintain bowel control. Take note if the patient's appetite decreases suddenly. It could indicate an underlying problem, such as a painful dental caries.

Elimination. Although the patient will eventually become incontinent as his illness progresses, take steps to maintain continence for as long as possible and to avoid urinary tract infections. Check on him frequently, staying alert for cues that he needs to void, such as restlessness or picking at clothes. If he's capable of using the toilet himself, label the door with bright colors and a picture of a toilet. If not, take him to the bathroom at least every 2 hours. Also note changes in his mental status, which could indicate constipation or a urinary tract infection.

Provide a high-fiber, high-fluid diet to prevent constipation. Eventually, the patient may have to switch from a regular diet to liquid supplements, increasing the risk of constipation or diarrhea. Monitor and record bowel function carefully. To prevent infection and decubitus ulcers, keep the skin clean and dry, use a condom catheter or indwelling catheter, and follow strict aseptic technique. If the patient shows signs of incontinence, assess for an underlying medical cause, such as an infection, an enlarged prostate, or fecal impaction.

Controlling agitation. The patient may behave inappropriately, pacing, cursing, screaming, biting, fighting, or wandering aimlessly. Don't discourage him from wandering—it stimulates circulation, decreases contracture formation, reduces stress, and provides a feeling of freedom. To protect him, put him in a room close to the nursing

Organic Mental Disorders

station, clear the area of as many hazards as possible, make sure he wears an identification bracelet, and provide hospital security with a recent photograph of him. Keep in mind that the wandering patient burns a lot of calories, so monitor his weight closely and provide extra calories, as needed.

Some agitated behaviors may prove difficult to accommodate or control. A patient may become excessively upset when confused or frightened (catastrophic reaction). For example, he may cry if you ask him a question he can't answer, or he may become combative when you assist him in the shower. Try to redirect his behavior. Distract him by suggesting a walk or a cup of tea, and give him a chance to calm down. Keep in mind that he doesn't know where he is or what's happening. To control anxiety, reassure him that you'll protect him from harm. Also assess whether his agitation may have an underlying physical cause, such as a reaction to medication.

If you have to use restraints, first identify the behavior you need to control. For example, the patient who paces constantly may require rest periods for at least 30 minutes every 4 hours. Ensuring rest may require you to restrain him with vest restraints in a bed or wheelchair. Vest restraints prevent falls and allow the patient's arms and legs to move freely. When the patient's in a wheelchair, make sure that he doesn't slide down and choke. If he's lying down, elevate the head of the bed to prevent choking, and turn him every 2 hours to prevent skin breakdown. While he's resting, elevate his legs to check for swelling and blisters.

Extremely agitated patients may need wrist restraints to prevent them from pulling out I.V.s, dressings, and catheters. To avoid contractures, cellulitis, or friction burns, use them only for short periods.

The doctor may order low doses of neuroleptics, such as haloperidol (Haldol) or thioridazine (Mellaril), to control agitation. Keep in mind that chlorpromazine (Thorazine) causes blood pressure to decrease more than other neuroleptics.

Providing care in pseudodementia. Patients with pseudodementia require the same interventions needed for other depressive disorders, including drug therapy with tricyclic antidepressants, monoamine oxidase inhibitors, or lithium carbonate. Monitor the patient for adverse effects and teach family members about them.

Encourage the patient to express his feelings. Listen attentively and allow for slow responses. To give him some control over his life, provide a structured routine with limited choices. For example, ask him if he'd like to shower before or after breakfast. Give simple instructions and write down important points. Encourage involvement in group activities to prevent isolation.

Help the patient with maintaining hygiene and with eating, as needed. Add high-fiber foods to his diet if he's constipated, and encourage physical activity. Be on the alert for increased despondency, and ask him directly if he's thought of hurting himself or of committing suicide. If the patient appears at risk for suicide, consult the doctor immediately, initiate precautions, and observe carefully. (For more information, see Chapter 4.)

Continued on page 154

Organic Mental Disorders

Dementias—*continued*

Managing MID. Interventions include preventing further strokes by controlling hypertension and other cardiovascular risk factors. Nursing measures may include teaching the importance of controlling weight, lowering dietary cholesterol, and quitting smoking. If his dementia isn't too severe, a patient with gait disturbance, hemiparesis, or speech and language problems may benefit from referral to a rehabilitation program. Behavior problems may require interventions similar to those for Alzheimer's patients. Refer to the results from the patient's mental status examination to find out his remaining strengths and skills and build on them.

Coping with extrapyramidal disorders. Interventions for Parkinson's disease include drug therapy with levodopa (Larodopa), amantadine (Symmetrel), or bromocriptine (Parlodel). These drugs increase cerebral dopamine function and may dramatically improve movement abnormalities. However, they're less successful in treating the dementia associated with Parkinson's disease.

Make the patient and his family aware of potential adverse effects from drug therapy. Levodopa may cause confusion or frequent involuntary choreic movements, amantadine may cause confusion, and bromocriptine may cause nightmares, hallucinations, or paranoid delusions. All three may cause hypotension. Take the patient's lying, sitting, and standing blood pressure, and instruct him to rise slowly from a sitting or lying position. Because drug effects wear off suddenly, administer each dose as close to the prescribed time as possible.

Look for ways to reduce the effects of the disorder and share them with the patient. For example, assess his ability to swallow, then recommend a diet that he can tolerate without choking. Prevent constipation by providing plenty of dietary fiber and liquids and by administering laxatives and enemas, as needed. Because the patient moves and thinks slowly, allow plenty of time for him to complete tasks; for example, bring him his food tray first and collect it last.

To help the patient cope with forgetfulness, write down key information. Observe what time of day the patient's at his best (usually when medication is at its peak effect), and plan your care and teaching accordingly. The patient may benefit from physical and speech therapy. Be especially alert for signs of severe depression or suicidal ideation.

Although no medical treatment can change the course of Huntington's disease, neuroleptic drugs, such as haloperidol, can decrease choreic movements. Patients with accompanying psychoses or mood disorders may receive additional drugs. Nursing measures include instruction on how to prevent and control choking, a persistent danger.

Combatting chronic confusional states. Prompt treatment may reverse chronic confusional states. Support the patient and family during treatment, and carefully monitor his condition and mental status to prevent relapse.

Helping families to cope. When the behavior and thinking of a loved one deteriorates, family members feel frightened, ashamed, de-

Organic Mental Disorders

pressed, and overwhelmed. Make providing support to family members an integral part of your nursing care. You can help provide the family with information on the course of illness, what behavior to expect from the patient, and available community resources.

Explain to family members that behaviors associated with irreversible dementia, such as memory loss and wandering, will worsen. Encourage use of safety measures at home; for example, having the patient wear an identification bracelet and placing locks on cabinets and doors.

Dealing with feelings. Family members often become angry when the patient begins to ask them to repeat what they've just said or is unable to live up to his former capabilities. When they realize the patient can't control his behavior, they usually experience guilt. They may also feel an overwhelming sense of loss upon realizing the patient will never return to his old self and that their relationship will never be the same. Let family members know such emotions are normal and encourage them to acknowledge their feelings. To help them regain some of their pride in the patient, take the time to ask what their loved one was like before his illness. Also recognize that family members might project some of their anger on you and your colleagues.

Planning care. Encourage family members to plan breaks from the routine involved in caring for the patient. Provide information on available home care agencies or day-care programs that may offer a source of relief. Discuss the possibility of placing the patient in a long-term care facility if his behavior worsens. Refer them to the hospital social worker to obtain a list of appropriate facilities. If the family decides to seek long-term care, help them cope with guilt and grief.

Refer family members to national and community resources, such as the Alzheimer's Disease and Related Disorders Association or the Huntington's Disease Foundation. Such organizations may enable family members to obtain support from individuals who share common experiences and may provide referrals for obtaining financial and legal assistance.

Families of patients with Alzheimer's disease and Huntington's disease may also ask for information on the hereditary nature of these disorders. Besides referring them to national and community-based sources of information, you may also make information on genetic inheritance part of family teaching. For example, you may explain to relatives of patients with Huntington's disease about the recently discovered genetic marker for the Huntington's disease gene. Help family members who want to be tested to make arrangements. If you learn of any relevant research studies that require volunteers, consider letting family members know. Emphasize that participating is strictly voluntary. It offers hope for some families but places increased stress on others.

Most dementia patients die in a medical setting from an acute infection. Discuss with families members their feelings about halting drastic resuscitation measures and preserving the patient's right to die with dignity. Make sure they understand all ethically sound

Continued on page 156

Organic Mental Disorders

Dementias—*continued*

options. After a patient's death, some family members may feel relieved, whereas others may feel grief-stricken. In either instance, family members will continue to need your support.

Finally, caring for a patient can be emotionally exhausting for you and your colleagues. So besides supporting the patient and family, support each other, especially by offering to relieve colleagues at regular intervals.

Evaluation

Base your evaluation on the patient's expected outcomes listed in the nursing care plan on page 151. To determine if the patient's needs are being met, ask yourself questions like these:
• Do others communicate with the patient at his level of ability?
• Does he follow directions when given appropriate cues?

The answers to these questions will help you assess your patient's status and the effectiveness of his care. Remember that these questions stem from the sample nursing care plan; your questions may differ.

Self-test

1. Causes of organic mental disorders may include all of the following except:
a. brain injury from head trauma   **b.** abuse of alcohol or psychoactive drugs   **c.** depression   **d.** primary disease of the brain

2. All of the following symptoms usually appear during the early stage of Alzheimer's disease except:
a. aphasia   **b.** suspicious delusions   **c.** a decline in computation skills   **d.** impaired remote memory

3. When assessing the patient with dementia, use the mental status examination to assess all of the following except:
a. awareness   **b.** the ability to distinguish reality from fantasy
c. the ability to understand spoken language   **d.** recent memory

4. Diffuse EEG slowing may indicate the patient has entered the early stages of degenerative dementia.
a. true   **b.** false

5. Which of the following is not recommended as an intervention for the patient with Alzheimer's disease?
a. low doses of neuroleptics to control agitation   **b.** use of plastic dishes and cups to avoid injury during mealtime   **c.** use of restraints if agitated behaviors cannot be controlled in other ways   **d.** offering a choice between two main courses at mealtimes to cultivate a feeling of independence

Answers (page number shows where answer appears in text)
1. **c** (page 142)   2. **b** (page 143)   3. **b** (page 147)   4. **b** (page 152)
5. **d** (page 152)

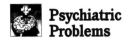

Selected References

Books

Alcoholics Anonymous. New York: Alcoholics Anonymous World Services, Inc., 1976.

American Nurses' Association and National Nurses Society on Addictions. *Standards of Addictions: Nursing Practice With Selected Diagnoses and Criteria.* Kansas City, Mo.: American Nurses' Association, 1987.

Benner, M. *Mental Health and Psychiatric Nursing: A Study and Learning Tool.* Springhouse, Pa.: Springhouse Corp., 1988.

Braun, B.G. *Treatment of Multiple Personality Disorders.* Washington, D.C.: American Psychiatric Association, 1986.

Burgess, A.W. *Psychiatric Nursing in the Hospital and the Community,* 4th ed. Englewood Cliffs, N.J.: Prentice Hall, 1985.

Carpenito, L.J. *Nursing Diagnosis: Application to Clinical Practice,* 2nd ed. Philadelphia: J.B. Lippincott Co., 1987.

Diagnostic and Statistical Manual of Mental Disorders, 3rd ed., revised. Washington, D.C.: American Psychiatric Association, 1987.

Haber, J., et al. *Comprehensive Psychiatric Nursing,* 3rd ed. New York: McGraw-Hill Book Co., 1987.

Hagerty, B.K. *Psychiatric–Mental Health Assessment.* St. Louis: C.V. Mosby Co., 1984.

Millon, T., and Everly, G.S. *Personality and Its Disorders: A Biosocial Learning Approach.* New York: John Wiley & Sons, 1985.

Murray, R.B., and Huelskoetter, M.M.W. *Psychiatric/Mental Health Nursing: Giving Emotional Care,* 2nd ed. East Norwalk, Conn.: Appleton & Lange, 1987.

Norris, J., et al. *Mental Health–Psychiatric Nursing: A Continuum of Care.* New York: John Wiley & Sons, 1987.

Rawlins, R.P., and Heacock, P.E. *Clinical Manual of Psychiatric Nursing.* St. Louis: C.V. Mosby Co., 1988.

Strub, R.L., and Black, F.W. *The Mental Status Examination in Neurology,* 2nd ed. Philadelphia: F.A. Davis Co., 1985.

Stuart, G.W., and Sundeen, S.J. *Principles and Practice of Psychiatric Nursing,* 3rd ed. St. Louis: C.V. Mosby Co., 1987.

Talbott, J.A., et al. *Textbook of Psychiatry.* Washington, D.C.: American Psychiatric Association, 1988.

Townsend, M.C. *Nursing Diagnoses in Psychiatric Nursing.* Philadelphia: F.A. Davis Co., 1988.

Wilson, H.S., and Kneisl, C.R. *Psychiatric Nursing,* 3rd ed. Menlo Park, Calif.: Addison-Wesley Publishing Co., 1988.

Periodicals

Cahill, C., and Arana, G.W. "Navigating Neuroleptic Malignant Syndrome," *American Journal of Nursing* 86(6):670-73, June 1986.

Dommisse, C.S., and Hayes, P.E. "Current Concepts in Clinical Therapeutics: Anxiety Disorders, Part I," *Clinical Pharmacy* 6(2):140-47, February 1987.

Dommisse, C.S., and Hayes, P.E. "Current Concepts in Clinical Therapeutics: Anxiety Disorders, Part II," *Clinical Pharmacy* 6(3):196-215, March 1987.

Folstein, M.J., et al. "Mini-Mental State: A Practical Method for Grading the Cognitive State of Patients for the Clinician," *Journal of Psychiatric Research* 12(3):189-98, November 1975.

Gallop, R. "The Patient is Splitting: Everyone Knows and Nothing Changes," *Journal of Psychosocial Nursing* 23(4):6-10, April 1985.

Jorgensen, P., and Munk-Jorgensen, P. "Patients with Delusions in a Community Psychiatric Service. A Follow-up Study," *Acta Psychiatrica Scandanavica* 73(2):191-95, February 1986.

Lucas, M.J., et al. "Recognition of Psychiatric Symptoms in Dementia," *Journal of Gerontological Nursing* 12(1):11-15, January 1986.

Rabins, P.V., et al. "The Impact of Dementia on the Family," *Journal of the American Medical Association* 248(3):333-35, July 1982.

Reich, P., and Gottfried, L. "Factitious Disorders in a Teaching Hospital," *Annals of Internal Medicine* 99(2):240-47, August 1983.

Saunders, J.M., and Valente, S.M. "Cancer and Suicide," *Oncology Nursing Forum* 15(5):575-81, September-October 1988.

Shapira, J., et al. "Distinguishing Dementias," *American Journal of Nursing* 86(6):698-702, June 1986.

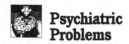

Index

i refers to an illustration; t refers to a table

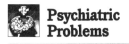

Index

i refers to an illustration; t refers to a table

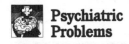
Index

i refers to an illustration; t refers to a table